Guide to Working
Europe for Doctor

For Churchill Livingstone:
Commissioning Editor: Timothy Horne
Project Development Manager: Janice Urquhart
Project Manager: Frances Affleck
Design direction: Erik Bigland
Illustrated by: Robin Dean from originals by K. E. A. Darling

Guide to Working in Europe for Doctors

K. E. A. Darling MB BS BSc(Hons) MRCP
Wellcome Clinical Training Fellow, Division of Infectious Diseases, Hammersmith Hospital, London, UK

FOREWORD BY
Professor Charles van Ypersele de Strihou
Departement de Nephrologie
Clinique Universitaires de Louvain
Brussels, Belgium

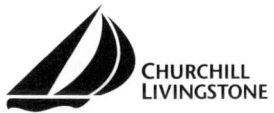

EDINBURGH LONDON NEW YORK PHILADELPHIA ST LOUIS SYDNEY TORONTO 2000

CHURCHILL LIVINGSTONE
An imprint of Harcourt Publishers Limited

© Harcourt Publishers Limited 2000

 is a registered trade mark of Harcourt Publishers Limited

The right of Katie Darling to be identified as author of this work has been asserted by her in accordance with the Copyright, Designs and Patents Act 1988.

All rights reserved. No part of this publication may be reproduced, stored in a retrieval system, or transmitted in any form by any means, electronic, mechanical, photocopying, recording or otherwise, without either the prior permission of the publishers (Harcourt Publishers Limited, 24–28 Oval Road, London NW1 7DX), or a licence permitting restricted copying in the United Kingdom issued by the Copyright Licensing Agency Ltd, 90 Tottenham Court Road, London, W1P 0LP UK.

First published 2000
ISBN 0 443 06281 1

British Library Cataloguing in Publication Data
A catalogue record for this book is available from the British Library.

Library of Congress Cataloging in Publication Data
A catalog record for this book is available from the Library of Congress.

Medical knowledge is constantly changing. As new information becomes available, changes in treatment, procedures, equipment and the use of drugs become necessary. The author and the publishers have, as far as it is possible, taken care to ensure that the information given in this text is accurate and up to date. However, readers are strongly advised to confirm that the information, especially with regard to drug usage, complies with current legislation and standards of practice.

The publisher's policy is to use **paper manufactured from sustainable forests**

Printed in China

Foreword

As long as the professional life of physicians was restricted to the country of origin, we failed to recognize how cumbersome and complicated our registration procedures were. At the end of medical school we followed en masse the common path unaware that a fresh look might find it tortuous.

Then came the European Community (now Union) regulations allowing the free movement of workers. Enthusiastic young doctors, eager to pursue their postgraduate training abroad, quickly discovered the complexity of the various national registration procedures. Trusting the claim that labour movement was free within the EC, the young Senior House Officer or equivalent, arriving in the host institution with his/her own national credentials, had then to chart a course in unknown territories to obtain the authorization to practise medicine in another member state of the Union. These pioneers quickly discovered that a variety of regulations had to be taken into account. Fortunately, most of them benefited from the help of senior physicians in whose department they were to be hosted.

Katie Darling had the same experience when leaving the UK for Belgium to spend a year of postgraduate training in internal medicine. As most pioneers, she was endowed not only with superb medical qualifications but also with other gifts one of which was the desire to help other junior physicians. She has an unusual ability to gather, classify and expose a wealth of information not only on registration procedures but also on the organization of postgraduate training in Europe.

This book offers a synthesis of all the information needed for junior applicants eager to experience the practice of medicine in the different member states. My guess would be that this endeavour is the first in its category. Had it been available in 1977 when the European exchange scheme for residents was initiated, the chiefs of medicine sitting in its steering committee would have saved a lot of time.

Katie's *Guide to Working in Europe for Doctors* is not only timely, it is also a testimony to the desire of European Physicians to achieve an integrated medical system for training as well as for health care delivery.

Professor Charles van Ypersele de Strihou
Belgium, Brussels

Preface

DO YOU SPEAK DUTCH AND CAN YOU INTUBATE?

Since 1977, it has been possible for doctors native to and trained in a country within the European Community to work in other member states without the need to sit local examinations. In the past 20 years, the Community has continued to tackle barriers to freedom of movement while at the same time embracing other countries as member states.

In many countries, medical education is changing so that doctors wishing to specialize must obtain a place on a recognized training programme before achieving specialist status. In Britain, this 'Calmanization', as it has become known, has led to a backlog of junior doctors waiting until more specialist training posts become available.

Increasing freedom of movement within the European Union, as it is now called, together with the longer period of time spent at pre-specialist level, has led to increasing numbers of junior doctors seeking employment abroad. This book is aimed at both these individuals and those of higher grades, as well as medical students and research workers who seek a 'European experience' to enhance the basic medical training enjoyed by the rest of their compatriots.

I had the opportunity to begin this book while preparing for a medical exchange post between a French-speaking Brussels teaching hospital and Hammersmith Hospital in London. At the time, there were no publications of reference and very limited information in general that provided the practical details I needed. I muddled through with the aid of tips from previous exchangees and hours of fruitlessly surfing on the Internet. The whole process was time-consuming and, on top of starting a new post in a new country in a second language, something I could have done without.

Administrative problems aside, the experience abroad was invaluable and gave me the inspiration to carry on writing. I was ideally placed, given that Brussels is the Babel of Europe. The information provided in each country chapter has been gathered with the help of certain colleagues who are native Danish, Greek, Spanish, German, Portuguese and Italian speakers. It was possible in this way to contact all medical associations or competent authorities that do not correspond in English, and to ensure the accuracy of my information.

PREFACE

Working in a different culture in a different health system is challenging and allows one to view one's home set-up in another light, for better or worse and often for both. The first 3 weeks abroad are gruelling and tiring but they pass and going on to tackle the next phase of obstacles starts to become rewarding instead of demoralizing. I have an anecdote which illustrates my point.

After 4 weeks on the wards in Brussels, I had reached the stage of speaking to patients and nurses, they understanding my questions and I their replies (just about). The time had come for my first night on call for Accident and Emergency and I approached the impending 24-hour shift with some trepidation. The staff there were friendly and welcoming, as was my supervisor. The latter introduced himself as he was leaving and muttered over his shoulder in French, 'By the way, Brussels is officially bilingual so you may need your Dutch and staff on call here have to cover the anaesthetists if they are busy with an emergency — are you OK with propofol?' The night passed, everyone spoke French, no one died and my doubtful anaesthetic skills were not called upon.

The question, 'Do you speak Dutch and can you intubate?, stayed with me as a metaphor for the never-ending obstacles that one encounters when working abroad. Just as matters come within reach of being under control, more problems are thrown in which need to be tackled. The rewards in the end are worth it, though, and I would recommend a stint abroad for anyone with a little determination, a lot of motivation and a reasonable sense of humour.

K. E. A. Darling   1999
London

Acknowledgements

This book has required extensive research from sources in each of the fifteen European Union member states and the countries of the European Economic Area. The following people and organizations have made the final compilation possible.

The national embassies, medical associations and competent authorities in Brussels and London. In Brussels, Professor van Ypersele de Strihou, Miss Karin Voss and, for her help with Danish and Greek translations, Dr Anna Chioti. Elsewhere, Dr Efrem Eren, Professor Gareth Williams, Dr Henry Bettinson and Dr Punit Ramrakha.

I would also like to thank Wendy Lee, who edited the final draft, for her linguistic expertise and tireless attention to detail.

Finally, my family and friends for their patience while I have been writing this book — in fact, for their patience in general.

Contents

How to use this book — xvii
Abbreviations and definitions — xxi

Section 1. General background — 1

1. About the European Union — 3
Brief history — 3
Administrative bodies of EU — 6
How legislation is passed — 7
Implications for health-care professionals — 8
Summary — 9

2. Differences between EU member states — 11
Europe by region — 11
Organization of health-care systems — 13
Education and clinical training — 16
Terms and conditions of employment — 17
Practical differences in the workplace — 18
Culture and ethics — 19

3. Moving abroad — practical points — 23
When to go — 23
Becoming registered and finding employment — 26
European schemes in action — 30
Cost — 33

Section 2. Country chapters — 41

4. Austria — 43
Background — 44
Language — 44
Organization of the health system — 44
Training and types of post — 45
Registration — 45

Finding a post 46
List of hospitals 46
Addresses 47
Registrable qualifications for Austrian doctors going abroad 48

5. Belgium 49
Background 49
Language 51
Organization of the health system 52
Training and types of post 54
Practical points 55
Registration 57
Finding a post 60
List of hospitals 61
Addresses 62
Registrable qualifications for Belgian doctors going abroad 63

6. Denmark 65
Background 65
Language 67
Organization of the health system 67
Training and types of post 68
Registration 69
Finding a post 69
List of hospitals 69
Addresses 71
Registrable qualifications for Danish doctors going abroad 71

7. Finland 73
Background 73
Language 75
Organization of the health system 75
Training and types of post 78
Practical points 78
Registration 79
Finding a post 81
List of hospitals 81
Addresses 82
Registrable qualifications for Finnish doctors going abroad 84

8. France 85
Background 85

Language	87
Organization of the health system	87
Training and types of post	92
Practical points	94
Registration	94
Finding a post	97
List of hospitals	97
Addresses	99
Registrable qualifications for French doctors going abroad	99
9. Germany	**101**
Background	101
Language	103
Organization of the health system	103
Training and types of post	106
Practical points	107
Registration	108
Finding a post	110
List of hospitals	111
Addresses	111
Registrable qualifications for German doctors going abroad	112
10. Greece	**115**
Background	115
Language	117
Organization of the health system	117
Training and types of post	119
Practical points	120
Registration	120
Finding a post	121
List of hospitals	121
Addresses	122
Registrable qualifications for Greek doctors going abroad	122
11. Republic of Ireland (Eire)	**125**
Background	125
Language	126
Organization of the health system	126
Training and types of post	129
Registration	129
Finding a post	130
List of hospitals	130

CONTENTS

    Addresses   131
    Registrable qualifications for Irish doctors going abroad   132

12. Italy   133
    Background   133
    Language   135
    Organization of the health system   135
    Training and types of post   137
    Practical points   138
    Registration   138
    Finding a post   138
    List of hospitals   139
    Addresses   139
    Registrable qualifications for Italian doctors going abroad   139

13. Luxembourg   141
    Background   141
    Language   143
    Organization of the health system   143
    Training and types of post   145
    Practical points   145
    Registration   146
    Finding a post   146
    List of hospitals   146
    Addresses   147
    Registrable qualifications for doctors from Luxembourg going abroad   147

14. The Netherlands   149
    Background   149
    Language   150
    Organization of the health system   151
    Training and types of post   154
    Practical points   155
    Registration   156
    Finding a post   156
    List of hospitals   157
    Addresses   158
    Registrable qualifications for Dutch doctors going abroad   159

15. Portugal   161
    Background   161

Language	163
Organization of the health system	163
Training and types of post	165
Practical points	166
Registration	166
Finding a post	166
List of hospitals	167
Addresses	168
Registrable qualifications for Portuguese doctors going abroad	168
16. Spain	**171**
Background	171
Language	173
Organization of the health system	173
Training and types of post	176
Practical points	177
Registration	178
Finding a post	178
List of hospitals	178
Addresses	179
Registrable qualifications for Spanish doctors going abroad	179
17. Sweden	**181**
Background	181
Language	183
Organization of the health system	183
Training and types of post	188
Practical points	188
Registration	189
Finding a post	190
List of hospitals	190
Addresses	191
Registrable qualifications for Swedish doctors going abroad	192
18. United Kingdom	**195**
Background	195
Language	197
Organization of the health system	198
Training and types of post	202
Practical points	204
Registration	206
Finding a post	208

List of hospitals	208
Addresses	210
Registrable qualifications for British doctors going abroad	211

19. Countries in the European Economic Area: Norway, Iceland and Liechtenstein — 213

Norway — 214
- Background — 214
- Language — 214
- Organization of the health system — 215
- Training and types of post — 215
- Addresses — 215
- Registrable qualifications for Norwegian doctors going abroad — 215

Iceland — 216
- Background — 217
- Language — 217
- Training and types of post — 217
- Addresses — 217
- Registrable qualifications for Icelandic doctors going abroad — 218

Liechtenstein — 218
- Background — 219
- Language — 219
- Training and types of post — 219
- Addresses — 219
- Registrable qualifications for doctors from Liechtenstein going abroad — 219

20. Switzerland — 221
- Background — 221
- Language — 222
- Organization of the health system — 223
- Training and types of post — 223
- Finding a post — 224
- List of hospitals — 224
- Addresses — 224
- Swiss doctors working in Britain — 226

How to use this book

This book has been divided into two main parts. Information on individual countries is provided in Section II but I would advise the reader to start with Section I, which provides an overview of some general aspects of working abroad and outlines the pitfalls of which to be wary.

Chapter 1 gives a short history of the origins of the present European Union, together with a brief description of the workings within the Union and their implications for health-care professionals. The chapter is of general interest for anyone considering work in another EU member state. For those not interested in history, the notes on legislation are useful, as the terms mentioned are increasingly entering professional vocabulary. The list of abbreviations and definitions on page xxi is also helpful for quick reference on that score.

Chapter 2 deals with certain aspects of health care that are easily taken for granted in one's native country. Topics such as health-service organization, hospital categories, the education and training of doctors, terms and conditions of employment, and culture and ethics are covered. Of these, health-service organization is particularly important, as the concepts of health care described here are later referred to in the country chapters of Section II. Defining terms such as 'gatekeeper' and 'competent authority' in Chapter 2 saves reiteration later on.

Chapter 3 provides comprehensive practical advice that should be digested before even considering a stint abroad. As well as pointers on when to go, there is information on the general procedures for registering as a doctor abroad and on finding a post. The information here is then expanded in each country chapter. European schemes currently in operation are also described in Chapter 3, namely, the European Exchange Scheme for junior doctors and the Erasmus/Socrates programme. The section on costs is particularly useful, as financial outlay is easily underestimated. The checklist on page 34 is for reference prior to departure.

Section II provides specific information on each EU member state. Countries have been listed alphabetically for simplicity and, it has to be said, political correctness. Each chapter is set out as follows:

- panel showing the country's basic statistics — main sources: Organization for Economic Cooperation and Development (OECD) and European Commission

- map
- brief background
- notes on languages spoken in the country, including the main dialects
- organization of the health system — includes health insurance, health-service funding, hospital types, hospital management and access to specialist care
- medical education, specialist training and types of post
- practical points — includes administrative tasks, and duties performed by other health-service professionals (such as nurses, social workers, etc.)
- how to obtain registration as a medical practitioner
- how to find a job
- list of hospitals
- useful addresses — for registration and for obtaining further information
- list of primary qualifications awarded nationally which are recognized for registration in other EU member states.

For each country chapter, I have tried to make the section on health-system organization as readable as possible. While I appreciate it is of marginal interest to those not in public health medicine, it is none the less very relevant to anyone practising in the particular member state. As described in Chapter 2, health-service organization has implications for doctors with respect to ward and outpatient administration. Certain professional duties vary between member states and it is important to be aware of the basic principles before starting work.

The number of hospitals listed varies for each country. For countries with fewer than ten medical schools, the teaching hospitals of each are listed. For the rest, either the main teaching hospitals or other large institutions are mentioned, or else details are given on how this information can be obtained. All hospitals which have taken part in the European Exchange Scheme (see p. 32) have been included.

Registrable qualifications for doctors who are natives of or who have trained in the country described are listed at the end of each chapter. In this way a doctor from, say, Finland knows what primary qualifications are required in order to work in say, Portugal. This can only be a general guide, however; precise details should be obtained from the relevant member state authority.

Although Iceland, Liechtenstein, Norway and Switzerland are not EU members, a brief section on each has been included in Section II. European Free Trade Association (EFTA) countries (the first three) are included in the EEC Directive on freedom of movement of health-care professionals between member states. Conditions for the recognition of qualifications and permission to work are consequently similar to those in the EU. This is not the case for Switzerland but the country has been included, as two Swiss hospitals have taken part in the European Exchange Scheme, hosting numerous junior doctors from EU member states.

It should be mentioned that the information provided here is not exhaustive. I have endeavoured to cover the most important aspects of each topic while at the same time avoiding the temptation to produce a glorified telephone directory. The information is none the less comprehensive and fully accurate at the time of writing. Reference sources for additional information have been provided where relevant.

This book aims to provide practical guidelines for doctors who plan to work in another country in a way that should allow excessive Net-surfing to be bypassed. I hope you will enjoy reading it.

Abbreviations and definitions

AFMS	Anglo-French Medical Society
BMA	British Medical Association
BMJ	British Medical Journal
CARMF	Caisse Autonome de Retraite des Médecins Français
CCST	Certificate of Completion of Specialist Training
Competent authority	National body responsible for recognition of a medical practitioner's primary qualification with a view to granting registration to practise as a healthcare provider (The competent authority in the UK is the GMC.)
CCU	Coronary care unit
DALF	Diplôme d'Études en Langue Française
DELF	Diplôme Approfondi de Langue Française
DFEE	Department for Education and Employment
DHA	District Health Authority
EAEC	See Euratom
EC	European Community
ECSC	European Coal and Steel Community
Ecu	European currency unit
EEA	European Economic Area
EEC	European Economic Community
EFTA	European Free Trade Association
EMU	Economic and Monetary Union
Erasmus	European community action scheme for mobility of university students
EU	European Union
Euratom	European Atomic Energy Community (also EAEC)
EURES	European Employment Service
Eurostat	European Community's statistical office
FAO	Food and Agriculture Organization (UN)
FHSA	Family Health Service Authority
Gatekeeper	Concept of medical practitioner of first contact in primary care (GP) having authority to determine whether further referral for a presenting patient is appropriate

GDP	Gross domestic product
GMC	General Medical Council
GNP	Gross national product
GP	General practitioner
IELTS	International English Language Testing System
INAMI	Institut National d'Assurance Maladie-Invalidité
ITU	Intensive treatment unit (intensive care)
Lingua	Action programme promoting foreign language competence in the community
MEP	Member of the European Parliament
MRCP	Membership of the Royal College of Physicians
MSF	Médecins sans Frontières
NACPME	National Advice Centre for Post-graduate Medical Education. An information and advice centre for overseas-qualified doctors who wish to undertake medical training in the UK
NHS	National Health Service
ODTS	Overseas Doctors Training Scheme
OECD	Organization for Economic Cooperation and Development
Overseas doctor	A doctor native to or trained in a country outside the EU or EEA
PLAB	Professional and Linguistic Assesment Board
PRHO	Pre-registration house officer
RHA	Regional Health Authority
SAMU	Service d'Aide Médicale Urgente
SEA	Single European Act
SHO	Senior house officer
Socrates	An EC action programme for cooperation in the field of education
SpR	Specialist registrar
TEA	Training and Employment Agency Northern Ireland
UCLES	University of Cambridge Local Examination Syndicate
UK	United Kingdom
UN	United Nations

SECTION 1

General background

About the European Union

BRIEF HISTORY

The origins of a united Europe date back to the early 1950s and the post-war years of economic depression. After two world wars, leaders of the countries of Western Europe were seeking a way to safeguard peace for the future, while promoting economic and social progress. A synopsis of events is shown in Box 1.1.

> **BOX 1.1**
> **Key events in the history of the European Union**
>
> | | |
> |---|---|
> | 1945 | End of Second World War |
> | 1951 | Treaty of Paris → ECSC |
> | 1957 | Treaty of Rome → EEC |
> | | Euratom |
> | 1960 | Stockholm Convention → EFTA |
> | 1973 | First expansion of EC, with joining of Denmark, UK and Ireland |
> | 1979 | First direct elections to European Parliament by universal suffrage |
> | 1986 | Signing of the Single European Act |
> | 1990 | Schengen Agreement |
> | 1992 | Treaty on European Union in Maastricht; led to EMU |
> | 1992 | EEA Treaty |
> | 1997 | A new Treaty for Europe, signed in Amsterdam |

It was Jean Monnet, French economist and public servant, who suggested an agreement between France and Germany to the French foreign minister Robert Schuman and the German Chancellor Konrad Adenauer. Proposals were drawn up by Monnet and Schuman in May 1950 for joint control of coal and steel production, two important industries at the time, between the two nations, and other countries were invited to participate. The Treaty of Paris, establishing the European Coal and Steel Community (ECSC) was eventually signed in April 1951 by France, Germany, Italy, Belgium, the Netherlands and Luxembourg.

The success of the ECSC led to plans for a common market, with trade in areas other than coal and steel. The Treaty of Rome was signed in March 1957, forming the European Economic Community (EEC), in which barriers to trade and services were removed. The European Atomic Energy Community (Euratom) was also established at this time, to develop nuclear energy for peaceful uses. The EEC and Euratom came into effect in 1958. In July 1967 the ECSC, EEC and Euratom were formally amalgamated and became jointly known as the European Community (EC) or European Communities, although the abbreviation EEC remained in common use.

Other European countries, led by the UK, took the initiative to organize their own free trade area and in January 1960 the European Free Trade Association (EFTA) was established between the UK, Austria, Denmark, Norway, Portugal, Sweden and Switzerland with the signing of the Stockholm Convention.

During the 10 years that followed, trade within the Economic Community increased sixfold, while EC trade with the rest of the world trebled. The common market became an attractive venture and other countries were invited to apply for membership. In January 1973, the EC expanded to take in Denmark, Ireland and the UK. These countries were later to be followed by Greece in 1981, Spain and Portugal in 1986, and Austria, Finland and Sweden in 1995 (see Box 1.2).

BOX 1.2
European Union member states and dates of joining

1957	France
	Germany
	Italy
	Belgium
	Netherlands
	Luxembourg
1973	Denmark
	United Kingdom
	Ireland
1981	Greece
1986	Spain
	Portugal
1995	Austria
	Finland
	Sweden

Until 1979, Members of the European Parliament (MEPs) were members of national parliaments delegated to represent their individual countries at Strasbourg. In June 1979, the first elections to the European Parliament took place by direct universal suffrage in each Union country, and these elections continue to be held every 5 years.

In 1986 the Single European Act was signed, amending several articles of the Treaty of Rome regarding voting procedures in the Council of Ministers, and enlarging the legislative powers of the European Parliament. The now-familiar blue flag with its circle of twelve gold stars became the official symbol at this time.

In February 1992, the Treaty on European Union was signed in Maastricht. With the Maastricht Treaty the EC, up until that point essentially based on economic affairs, was transformed into a European Union, standing on three pillars:

- the European Community
- common foreign and security policy
- justice and home affairs.

The first pillar embraced the three existing European Community treaties (ECSC, EC and Euratom). The latter two pillars had hitherto been regarded as matters dealt with by the national governments.

The signing of the Maastricht Treaty marked the first time that issues surrounding health were considered as being part of a united responsibility. The Treaty also served to promote freedom of movement of individuals of any background between member states. Prior to this, such movement had been limited to regulated professions. Efforts at harmonization and mutual recognition of educational and professional qualifications between different member states are presently under way. What the Maastricht Treaty is also famous for is the decision on Economic and Monetary Union (EMU). This took effect on 1 January 1999 within member states that satisfied economic criteria. (The UK would have been eligible but opted out of this clause.)

Other agreements

The European Economic Area (EEA) Treaty was signed in 1992, but rejected in a referendum in Switzerland. When it came into force in January 1994, it included Iceland, Norway, Austria, Finland and Sweden. Liechtenstein joined later after revising economic relations with Switzerland; Austria, Finland and Sweden left to join the EU in 1995.

The Schengen Agreement was an initiative taken outside the EC framework by Germany, France and the Benelux countries in 1990. The Agreement established freedom of movement for individuals between countries within the 'Schengen Area'. Other countries have since joined the Agreement but the UK and Ireland continue to decline inclusion, wishing to retain control over who enters their territory. The Schengen Agreement was incorporated into the new Treaty for Europe, signed in Amsterdam in 1997.

This Treaty was ratified by the leaders of all 15 member states and has four main objectives:

- dealing with employment and citizens' rights
- ensuring freedom of movement
- directing Europe's role in world affairs
- enlarging the Union by accepting further European states as members.

ADMINISTRATIVE BODIES OF THE EU

European administration is dealt with by five main institutions:

1. *The European Commission* is based in Brussels and serves to propose new laws, to manage common EU policies and to organize their implementation in each member state. It is organized into 25 Directorates-General which deal with all policy areas. The Commission comprises 20 Commissioners appointed by the national governments of each member state. There are two Commissioners from each of the larger countries and one from each of the smaller ones.

2. *The Council of Ministers* is also based in Brussels and works to discuss proposals put forward by the European Commission. The Council ensures representation of national interests, amends proposals accordingly and decides whether or not the proposals should become law. The Council comprises government ministers from each member state. *The Economic and Social Committee* is a purely advisory body which must be consulted by the European Commission and the Council of Ministers over a wide range of issues.

3. *The European Parliament* is also consulted on proposals from the European Commission and in some cases jointly decides on legislation with the Council of Ministers. The Parliament comprises 626 MEPs elected from each member state by universal suffrage every 5 years. Parliament meets in Strasbourg for 1 week per month in plenary session. Its 20 specialist committees then meet in Brussels, where some plenary sessions are also held.

4. *The European Court of Justice* is based in Luxembourg and serves to interpret the Community's decisions and the provisions of the Treaty in the event of dispute. There are 15 judges from each member state, nominated by the Council of Ministers, and 9 Advocates-General.

5. *The Court of Auditors* is also based in Luxembourg; it monitors all financial transactions in the EU and publishes reports on financial management on behalf of tax-paying citizens. There are 15 members, one from each member state.

The European Council or summit comprises the Heads of State or Government of each member state. The Council usually meets twice a year to give overall direction to EU developments.

HOW LEGISLATION IS PASSED

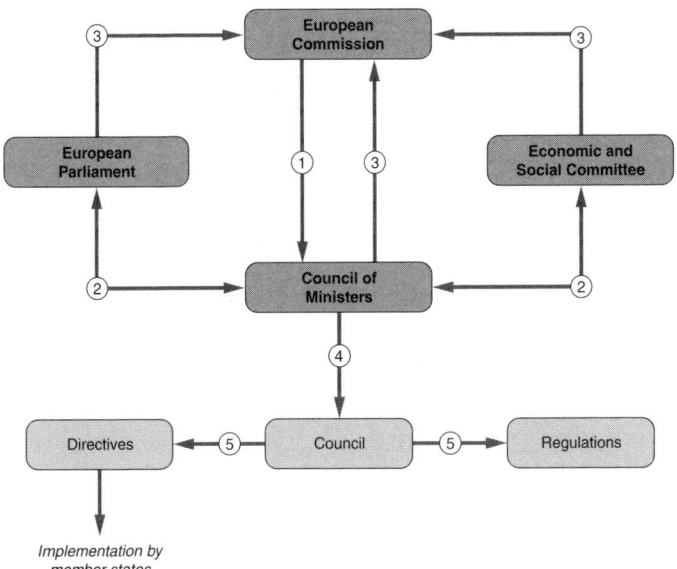

- Legislation is undertaken through regulations and directives. Proposals for legislation are initiated by the European Commission and adopted by the Council of Ministers. ①
- The Council then amends these proposals, in consultation with the European Parliament and the Economic and Social Committee. ②
- The Council then provides the Commission with the opportunity to amend the proposals, with opinions from the Parliament and the Economic and Social Committee. ③ Amended proposals are then reviewed by the Council. ①
- This loop continues until the final proposal is accepted and a decision is made. ④
- Legislation is then undertaken in the form of regulations and directives, ⑤ the latter then being implemented by the EU member states (see text).

Fig. 1.1 How European legislation is passed.

Glossary of terms

Community legislation adopted by the Council of Ministers or by the Council and the European Parliament in co-decision procedures may take the following forms:

- *regulations* — laws that are binding and apply to all member states, overriding national law
- *directives* — laws that are binding and lay down compulsory objectives, although the means of achieving these is left to national authorities
- *decisions* — laws that are binding in all their aspects but only to the member states, companies or individuals to whom they are addressed
- *recommendations* — and *opinions* — statements not laws; they are not binding.

IMPLICATIONS FOR HEALTH-CARE PROFESSIONALS

The development of the EU has enabled health-care professionals to work in any member state without the need for a work permit. Residence permits are still required, however; any individual from an EU member state must apply for one but will automatically receive it if moving to another state within the EU.

The recognition of doctors' diplomas was first tackled in 1975, the EEC issuing two directives concerning medical qualifications and training. The first directive dealt with the mutual recognition of primary medical qualifications and specialist medical qualifications for individuals from and training in EU member states. The second directive dealt with the minimum standards of training required in order to be awarded such qualifications. Mutual recognition came into effect in 1977. In 1986 this was extended to include vocational training of GPs, and both the 1977 and 1986 directives were superseded in 1993 by Directive 93/16/EC.

It should be mentioned that, although recognition of primary qualifications is a huge step in tackling obstacles to freedom of movement, obtaining registration once abroad does not then guarantee a post in practice. Once registered, however, one is in theory just as eligible to apply for posts in the new member state as doctors who are native and who have trained there.

In 1990, member states agreed to extend the right of residence to students, pensioners and non-employed people, provided they have sufficient means to support themselves and have adequate health insurance cover. It was also recognized that job-seekers might also need time to look for work and so social security benefits were consequently extended to them. In this way, health-care professionals moving to other states can bring their spouses and children without the need for special permits.

SUMMARY

The EU now consists of 15 member states with a total population of 370 million people speaking 11 official languages. As barriers to movement are progressively being tackled and as communication systems such as the Internet expand, employment opportunities are increasingly available. As well as different cultures and languages, the EU provides a diversity of medical experience that is highly valuable to overall training and access to it continues to be facilitated.

For further details on the rights of EU citizens moving to other member states and for other general information, the following sources are useful:

Office of the European Parliament in London
European Parliament — Information Office
2 Queen Anne's Gate
London SW1H 9AA
Tel: 0171 227 4300
Fax: 0171 227 4302

Commission Representatives and Office in England
Jean Monnet House
8 Storey's Gate
London SW1P 3AT
Tel: 0171 973 1992
This office publishes a booklet entitled 'The European Union — What's in it for me?' which is full of practical information for anyone planning a move to another member state.

Information on the EU is available on the Internet and can be accessed through the Europa server at: http://europa.eu.int

Differences between EU member states

EUROPE BY REGION

This book is comprehensive but not exhaustive. The 'Background' section of each country chapter is brief and provides only salient points for the visitor. It has been assumed the reader has some insight into his or her chosen member state with respect to culture, lifestyle and practicalities. Details regarding health-service organization have been included, as these are relevant for medical practice but are not always immediately apparent and can be difficult to obtain. The following is a brief synopsis of the countries covered in Section II and is intended to supplement the individual chapters.

English-speaking countries (UK and Republic of Ireland)

These countries are popular for visiting doctors, as English is a common second language for the majority of continental European countries. Anglophone medicine is held in high regard with its emphasis on clinical technique, epitomized by the Membership examination of the various Royal Colleges (see p. 203). The UK is particularly popular with doctors trained in Germany and Greece (see Fig. 18.2, p. 198) and with citizens of non-EEA countries. The British Council in Manchester has an advice centre for EEA- and non-EEA-trained doctors who wish to work in the UK, and the British Medical Association (BMA) international department issues some useful information sheets. The latter is also a useful source for British nationals going abroad. (See p. 210 for address.)

Benelux countries (Belgium, the Netherlands and Luxembourg)

Belgium and the Netherlands have been regular hosts to British and other junior doctors as part of the European Exchange Scheme. The standard of training and medicine in general is high and the health systems are well developed. Belgium, home of the EC, is no stranger to bureaucracy and form-filling for incoming professionals is an exhausting but unavoidable part of life. Luxembourg has no medical school and so no teaching hospital as such, but operates a high standard of care none the less.

Work experience in Belgium and the Netherlands is usually acknowledged as part of general training on return to one's native land. Some visitors find certain ethical issues in the Netherlands — for example, Dutch views on euthanasia — difficult to become accustomed to at first (see below).

Remember that the working day in Belgian teaching hospitals can be long and that out-of-hours duty is unpaid. Hours per week are fewer in the Netherlands but consequently pay is lower.

French-speaking countries (France, Belgium, Switzerland and Luxembourg)

France is very accessible for British doctors, geographically and also linguistically, as French is the most common second language taught in British schools. There are other ties with French doctors by way of organizations such as the Anglo-French Medical Society and Médecins sans Frontières (MSF) (see p. 99). Having a base in francophone medicine is also useful for work in parts of Africa, Indochina and South America. French-speaking doctors can also work in Belgium, Switzerland and Luxembourg.

German-speaking countries (Germany, Austria, Switzerland and Luxembourg)

The health system in Germany, along with all other aspects of life, has undergone considerable change since unification in 1990. Medical unemployment and underemployment are high and many German-qualified doctors travel abroad to continue their training. The standard of medical practice in former West Germany is considered high. From the curriculum vitae viewpoint, work in this area would be regarded more highly at present than work in former East Germany or Austria, although health care and training in both the latter are expanding and rapidly improving. German-speaking doctors can also work in Switzerland and Luxembourg.

Norden

This term is used to cover the five countries situated in northern Europe: namely, Denmark, Finland, Iceland, Norway and Sweden. The Nordic countries have strong economic and political links. Their policies are co-ordinated by way of the Nordic Council, which was formed in 1952, and this has resulted in the harmonization of regulations and a free labour market.

The countries are ethnically homogeneous, especially Denmark, Norway and Sweden, although there are important minority groups, in particular the Saami (Lapp) populations and increasingly immigrants, particularly refugees.

The countries have large welfare state programmes and because of the similarity of their policies, medical education and training are fairly uniform. Doctors from these countries can move more freely within Norden than between their native country and other EU member states. Doctors from Denmark and Sweden can move between the two countries without obtaining equivalence of their qualifications.

The national medical associations are well organized and English is almost universally spoken by administrative officials (perhaps less so in Finland). The medical associations and competent authorities also provide comprehensive information on the national codes of practice, including ethical and legal issues. In some cases, the incoming doctor must be examined on these. The standard of health care, particularly in the EU states of Norden, is considered high.

Southern Europe (Spain, Portugal, Italy and Greece)

These countries give the impression of being less well organized as far as competent authorities and medical associations are concerned. Correspondence can be slow and it is advisable to have a contact on site to tackle the necessary administration and to deliver the relevant documents. I found the Spanish Embassy in London particularly helpful but other embassies less so. Unemployment and underemployment are also considerable, and Spain and Greece have the highest doctor-to-patient ratios in Europe. Training in these countries is held in lower regard than in countries further north and this is relevant in terms of one's curriculum vitae and future employment. Those aspects aside, the weather is great and the lifestyle is enviable.

Switzerland

Switzerland is not part of the EEA but nevertheless is a popular destination for all professional groups. Medical standards are high and employment is possible for French, German and Italian speakers. The main downside is the administration for registration and training for non-Swiss nationals. There is no recognition of equivalent grades from other EU member states and work permits and language tests are usually required. The European Exchange Scheme is an excellent way around this problem, and as the exchange post is for 6–12 months, the issue of training recognition is less important.

ORGANIZATION OF HEALTH-CARE SYSTEMS

Health-care systems differ and Box 2.1 summarizes the main types encountered in Europe. Government money spent on health care also varies,

> **BOX 2.1**
> **Health-care systems and hospital set-ups in Europe**
>
> **Health systems**
> - National health services
>   — State
> - Insurance-based
>   — Premiums paid by employer and employee
>   — Compulsory and voluntary (complementary) programmes
>   — Inpatient treatment paid directly to hospital by third-party insurance body payment
>   — Any payment up front by patient is later reimbursed by insurance body
>
> **Hospitals**
> - Public
>   — Income from State
> - Private
>   — Income from patients / insurance body +/− subsidy from State
>   For-profit — Income from patient charges +/− bank loans
>   Not-for-profit — Funds from charitable bodies / religious orders

although as can be seen in Figure 2.1 this is usually proportional to a country's gross domestic product (GDP).

Types of health system

National health services are funded by the State and health care is free to all

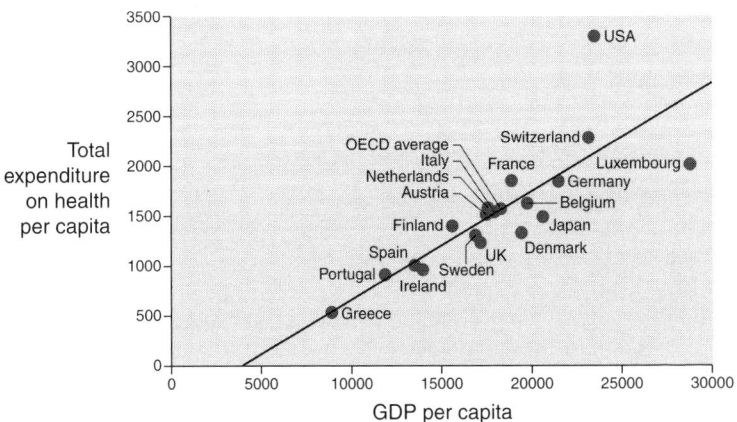

Fig. 2.1 Spending on health care versus gross domestic product (GDP) in Europe, the US and Japan. Calculated in Purchasing Power Parities in US dollars from OECD data (1993).

native citizens at the point of delivery. Co-payments are sometimes required in the form of either a set nominal fee or a small percentage of total cost for certain items such as prescription drugs, appliances and dental and optician services, except in the case of exemptions — for example, the elderly, disabled and unemployed.

Insurance-based health systems are more common and involve nationwide compulsory health insurance. Again, certain underprivileged groups are exempt or their insurance premiums are reduced and in most countries there are additional public, State-funded institutions for patients who cannot pay. Either payment for consultations, investigations and treatment is made directly to the health-service provider by the insurance body or else the patient pays part or all of the cost up front and is later reimbursed. Reimbursement varies according to indication for the care provided. Life-saving treatment is reimbursed at 100% whereas certain outpatient consultations and some prescription costs are reimbursed only in part. Some drugs have certain conditions for reimbursement — for example, H_2-antagonists require a copy of an endoscopy report confirming oesophagitis/gastritis/ulceration, and ACE inhibitors for hypertension require failure of other agents or satisfaction of other criteria. This has implications for the practising doctor, as patients will require proof that treatments are justified medically in order to be reimbursed. The doctor must therefore be prepared to complete insurance forms for inpatient treatment and be aware when prescribing of the different categories of pharmaceuticals and the conditions for reimbursement. These policies may seem bizarre to incoming doctors used to other systems but compliance with local administration is necessary to ensure payment for health-care providers.

Hospitals

Private and public hospitals exist throughout Europe, although in different proportions. Private hospitals are more numerous in countries with insurance-based health systems. With these systems, money for inpatient care moves with the patient as hotel costs and investigations are paid third-party by his or her insurance body. In this way, more ultrasound scanning or computed tomography per patient means more money paid to the hospital. As a result, investigations are performed more frequently than in government hospitals, where any additional procedures are a further drain on state resources.

Gatekeeping and the role of specialists

There are also differences in patient access to specialist care. In the UK, general practitioners have a '*gatekeeping*' role, whereby all patients must first present to them before they can be considered for specialist referral. In other countries, patients can present to any physician of their choice as often as they like, in the outpatient setting; admission to hospital still requires referral. In France, particularly, the phenomenon of 'medical nomadism' exists, whereby patients make multiple consultations with a variety of specialists, with subsequent reimbursement for the cost of each clinic visit. Lack of generalist gatekeeping can be expensive if the system is abused in this way and a degree of insight is required on the part of the patient. For example, should a patient with hypertension present to a cardiologist, a nephrologist, a specialist in general internal medicine or a clinical pharmacologist?

The other difference is at doctor level. It is possible and commonplace in certain countries for specialists to practise independently outside the hospital setting. A cardiologist, for example, may set up a clinic with electrocardiogram and echo facilities, provided he or she has attained specialist status. Equally, a hospital consultant may manage the general medical care of a patient who does not have a general practitioner and in this way serve as a primary-care provider in a secondary or tertiary environment.

EDUCATION AND CLINICAL TRAINING

Entry into study and selection processes

Medical schools in most countries have a *numerus clausus* or numerical limit on the number of places awarded. This limit can be related to anticipated manpower needs, as in Denmark and the UK, or to the educational capacity of medical schools, as in Germany, Ireland and the Netherlands. The *numerus clauses* can apply at entry, as in the UK, or later on — for example, at the end of the first year in France or the third year in Belgium. Italy has only recently introduced a limit on intake, and in Greece it is possible to bypass the system by doing pre-clinical studies elsewhere and then joining in for the clinical course.

For number limitation at entry, selection is based either on grades on leaving school, on time spent waiting for a place (in Germany) or on a national examination (the *selectividad* in Spain, the results of which are combined with school grades). Often these selection criteria are accompanied by a formal or informal interview.

Training

Training in most places in divided into pre-clinical and clinical parts. The amount of clinical teaching is very variable, however, and time spent on clinical skills is greater in the UK and Ireland than anywhere else. Qualified doctors in the UK are obliged to take medical students during the working day for 'bedside' teaching, where they watch the students examine patients and correct their technique.

Following final examinations, some countries have an internship period before full registration as a medical practitioner is awarded (see Box 2.2).

BOX 2.2
Internships in European countries

Internship	No internship
• Belgium	• Austria
• Greece	• Denmark
• Luxembourg	• Finland
• Netherlands	• France
• Spain	• Germany
• Switzerland	• Iceland
• UK	• Ireland
	• Italy
	• Liechtenstein
	• Norway
	• Portugal
	• Sweden

Further training differs with respect to how much time is spent in general medical training before training as a specialist begins. The UK and Ireland are the only countries which require Membership of one of the Royal Colleges before a doctor can begin specialization. Specialist training takes between 4 and 6 years, depending on specialty. Training programmes are limited in the UK and France according to anticipated specialist requirements. Entry on to a training programme can be very competitive and entry requirements are variable. Only Germany, Italy and Greece have exit examinations before specialist status is awarded, but in other countries logbooks documenting experience are required.

As discussed below, the range of specialist duties is not uniform between countries, and in places where specialization begins early in training, practical procedures are performed only by the relevant specialist.

TERMS AND CONDITIONS OF EMPLOYMENT

Hours and salary

Hours of work and salary are very variable between countries and even between regions, and both should be established before accepting any post. Working hours also vary between academic institutions and district general hospital equivalents. In Belgium, as mentioned, on-call duty is not paid, although paradoxically this can make doctors less aware of time spent after hours; there is little point in constantly watching the clock (arguably) if there is no reimbursement for extra duty. As we will see in Chapter 3, it is important to establish which country is providing the salary in the case of exchange arrangements, as a drop in salary is only one of many costs incurred when moving abroad.

Practical duties

In different countries, the duties of various clinical specialties can differ. For example, the responsibilities of gynaecologists extend to breast surgery in some countries, whilst in others this is dealt with by general or breast surgeons. In some of the larger teaching hospitals, practical procedures become segregated according to specialty so that chest physicians are called to aspirate pleural effusions, neurologists perform lumbar punctures and patients are sent to an anaesthetist if they require a central line.

PRACTICAL DIFFERENCES IN THE WORKPLACE
Language

Having a grasp of the local language is important for general communication but specialist vocabulary is also necessary. Local terms and phrases can then be acquired — for example, *un bon* is the French term for a blood or X-ray request form. Abbreviations are universal in medicine, whatever the language. (Try translating, 'Previous MI and CVA with SOB caused by LVF or PE' into another language for practice and see how long it takes.)

Nurses

Nursing skills differ widely and it is important to ascertain what nursing duties are. In some mainland European countries, nurses do everything from making beds and giving medication to taking blood, measuring arterial blood gases and performing electrocardiograms. In others, the general level of training is low and tasks such as intravenous drug administration belong to the duty doctor.

Drugs

Drug names do not differ very widely, given the linguistic differences between member states. What is likely to change, however, is the pronunciation or the fact that trade names rather than generic names are used. Formularies often list drugs alphabetically rather than according to drug family and this can cause difficulties with drugs that are specific to certain countries. Note also that culture is important with respect to prescribing. In francophone countries, for example, the rate of benzodiazepine prescribing is high, with little counselling regarding dependence. Certain nationalities expect treatment to be prescribed as a matter of course and telling the patient why it is not indicated goes down badly. This may explain the number of drugs of uncertain function available in some places.

Diseases

As demography differs between member states so does pathology. Certain conditions are more prevalent in some parts of Europe than others — for example, cardiovascular disease or certain infectious agents — and socio-economic factors and access to health care also play a role. Disease interpretation and cultural factors are also important. Having an understanding of these is as much a part of overall patient management as is performing blood tests and X-rays.

CULTURE AND ETHICS

Despite moves towards a 'united Europe', there are some aspects of life, such as climate, history, culture and religion, which can never change and will remain diverse throughout the continent. These aspects have implications for medical practice and a few examples are illustrated here.

Resuscitation status

This has many links with religious belief. The pro-life stance of Roman Catholicism is incompatible with the idea of allowing someone to die, regardless of prognosis. Thus in areas with a predominantly Catholic population, every patient tends to be for resuscitation unless the patient or family has explicit wishes to the contrary. Discussing resuscitation issues can be a taboo area. Considering every patient to be for resuscitation obviates the need for this discussion, while giving the impression of doing everything possible to keep the person alive.

Termination of pregnancy

Legislation on termination varies between countries and again is influenced by religious denomination. Details are available from the national competent authority. Note that in certain member states, involvement with other health-care professionals or persons of authority is required before termination can proceed.

Paternalism

In the context of health care, this is the idea of limiting a patient's freedom of knowledge, choice or both, for what is believed to be in his or her best interests. This has implications regarding the information that is imparted to a patient and so affects decision-sharing and consent.

In paternalistic cultures, a patient may not be told he or she has cancer, for example, but that there are 'bad' or 'malignant' cells. Doctors in this environment can argue that for some patients it is in their best interests not to know 'the full story'. Indeed, some degree of paternalism is exercised by many health-care professionals in certain situations. For example, it could be argued that patients who have a below-average level of intelligence do not need to be 'burdened' with knowledge of certain rare side-effects of a given drug if the benefits of this treatment sufficiently outweigh the risks. Here is not the place for ethical debate but, whatever one's beliefs, care should be taken that they are compatible with local legislation. In this way, information regarding the diagnosis of terminal illness must be considered in relation to policies on insurance and life assurance. Giving patients selective information might affect their position with regard to these policies.

Consent

This is linked to paternalism. In some countries, notably Belgium, consent is not required for post-mortem examination or HIV testing. In other countries consent is required for the latter as taking this test has implications for insurance. While obtaining consent, the health-care professional can use the opportunity to counsel the patient regarding risk behaviour and mode of infection transmission. Consent forms for invasive investigations and operations are also not universal.

Euthanasia

This represents the other extreme of the ethical issues discussed so far. In the Netherlands, the 'living will' was made legal in 1992 (see p. 155). This requires the complete passage of information between doctor and patient and an ability to broach the taboo subject of death. Many doctors who have trained elsewhere feel uncomfortable when first exposed to this system of management. Being aware of these issues in advance will help visiting doctors to deal with them and so be able to discuss them with patients.

Demography

Other cultural factors depend on the socio-economic profile of the patient population. This will affect education, returning to the idea of paternalism, and also the baseline standard of health. Poorer populations often have reduced access to primary health care owing either to fewer resources or to lack of patient awareness. In countries with insurance-based health care, doctors working in non-public institutions may be blissfully unaware of an area's true demography.

Socio-economic profile also affects the perceived status of health-care professionals — that is, whether doctors are regarded as knowledgeable authority figures or simply as people providing a service. Again, in insurance-based systems where patients are paying for their health care and have the freedom to move from doctor to doctor, the attitude is very much one of shopping for the best service available.

Common ground

Whatever the cultural, socio-economic and other differences, certain features of life are common to all countries. All EU member states have statistics for their growing elderly populations, disability, poverty and unemployment. Diseases such as ischaemic heart disease, cancer and HIV (with or without associated drug dependence or prostitution) are universal, although of varying prevalence. Concepts such as hospital management and quality assurance have had their profiles raised in the quest to improve health-service economy, and continuing medical education is being promoted as part of clinical training harmonization.

It is worth remembering these areas of common ground while being lost among the differences, as it helps to put matters into perspective. Focusing on points that are familiar will help the visitor realize that there is less to get used to than he or she might first have imagined.

Moving abroad — practical points

WHEN TO GO

Planning a move abroad will depend on personal and professional events and there may not be one particular 'best time' for everyone. There are, however, *better* times; the issues at each stage of training are discussed here.

The length of time spent abroad is also a factor to consider. For short-term posts, the stage of training and the chosen country probably matter less. For longer periods, points such as training programmes, equivalency of specialist status and health-care organization in general become more important, and the timing of the move abroad and the choice of country both require careful consideration.

The following information is based on the British training hierarchy but each level is defined with respect to years post-qualification so that it is meaningful to doctors from all member states.

Medical student (undergraduate)

Sabbaticals in Europe for medical students usually apply to the clinical stage (second half) of training. The two main options available depend on the length of study envisaged. The *Erasmus/Socrates* project is for periods of 6–12 months (see p. 30). Stays have to be planned well in advance and organization needs to involve both the student's native university and that of the host country. Most academic institutions in the UK have a European Liaison Officer who can advise on these projects but some centres are more *au fait* with the system than others. The faculty of medicine at the University of Liverpool is particularly pro-active and a number of successful exchanges with French-speaking institutions have taken place and continue to do so.

For shorter periods and for visits that can be organized individually, perhaps at shorter notice, there is the *medical elective*. Between the months of November and April, electives to France are popular as they tie in well with the skiing season and French is a common second language for many EU citizens. The elective period provides one of the best opportunities to visit a country, enjoy its culture and work in a foreign language, whilst avoiding such aspects as competent authority registration and medical responsibility. I would make the most of it.

Pre-registration house officer (PRHO or internist)

This is the period spent as a practising doctor, usually post-qualification, that is required before full registration with the national competent authority can be granted.

Once a student has completed medical studies, it is advisable to finish the PRHO year or equivalent in the country of study and obtain full registration before going further afield. Without having full registration in one country, it is difficult to be registered elsewhere. In some member states, an incoming doctor planning to stay and specialize may be required to work as a PRHO equivalent before training on a specialty programme can begin, even if he or she has full registration in the country of origin.

Senior house officer (SHO)

This is the period of general training spent after obtaining full registration with the national competent authority and before commencing a specialty training programme. In some countries, this stage does not exist as a separate entity but is considered as the first 1–2 years of a specialist programme.

This is a very good time to work abroad. It is beneficial for general training to work in a variety of specialist departments and there is less responsibility assigned at this level of training than later on. It is also a period when doctors are less likely to have personal commitments such as partners and children, and so have more freedom to travel.

The European Exchange Scheme is particularly directed at SHO level and some London teaching hospitals have incorporated a 6- or 12-month attachment abroad into their 2-year rotation schemes. This has the advantage of offering a post in Europe while providing job security on return home. One of the difficulties otherwise is that while a doctor is working abroad, it is not always possible to keep abreast of job vacancies at home. Returning for interviews is expensive and travel expenses are not reimbursed.

For British doctors, going away at SHO level can cause problems with respect to Membership (see p. 203). It is difficult to sit the examinations without the relevant teaching, and attending courses while away is really not feasible. One way round this is to obtain Membership first and then work abroad while waiting for a Calman National Training Number (NTN). In this way, one is in a better bargaining position on return than someone leaving midway through the SHO period who has the prospect of both Membership *and* job-hunting to come back to.

Specialist registrar (SpR)

This is the period of specialist training lasting between 4 and 6 years, undertaken with a view to becoming a consultant.

There are moves to unify specialist training in all EU member states. This is not yet the case, however, and so work experience in some states is not always recognized as part of specialist training in others. It is therefore vital that recognition is acknowledged *in writing* by the relevant body in charge of training *before* taking up the post. This cannot be stressed strongly enough.

Again, the duration of the visit is relevant. At any stage of specialist training, 6 or 12 months spent doing other things do not markedly alter training as a whole. If the period abroad is longer than this, or if the doctor plans to complete a specialist training programme in the country in question, then he or she may be required to work at a more junior level for 1 or 2 years before being eligible to start training as a specialist. In many countries gaining a place on a specialist training programme is highly competitive and there is considerable unemployment and underemployment. This is covered in more detail in the relevant country chapters.

Another important factor at SpR level is language. Doctors at this stage in training are assigned more responsibility and have junior colleagues to oversee. It is therefore vital to be able to communicate with patients, laboratory technicians and colleagues on the ward satisfactorily. Vocabulary for describing how to perform practical procedures is often overlooked but should be ready in case of crisis.

Consultant

This is the position awarded once specialist training has been completed. Such a doctor retains the title 'consultant' but may be promoted to head of department (chief consultant within a specialist division) or clinical director (in charge of all specialties within a given health-care institution).

The ease of moving abroad at this level depends on type of practice, be it hospital-based or work as an independent practitioner. If completion of specialist training can be recognized, a doctor can set up business privately once registration has been obtained and any other red tape (as for any private enterprise) has been tackled. Employment is then determined by market forces. Setting up practice can be a gamble, as it is often not easy to arrange and can result in salary cuts. Indeed, many would be unwilling to take such a gamble, having worked hard to obtain consultant status at home.

For hospital doctors, *exchange posts* are possible if a colleague at a similar level in the country of choice agrees and can be made available for the required period of time. In academic institutions, this can be arranged under the Socrates initiative (see p. 30) if the consultants in question are readers or professors (that is, in a teaching capacity). Exchanges of this type bypass the need for job-hunting, as both posts are already created. This is relevant, as finding permanent posts at this level is increasingly difficult wherever one applies.

General practitioners (GPs)

This term refers to doctors who work in primary care in the community or who are generalists in independent practice.

With the revised EEC Directive on mutual recognition of medical diplomas of 1986, GPs must complete 2–3 years' vocational training before being awarded specialist status (specialist in general medicine). If planning to practice abroad, a GP may be required to work for 1–2 years as a hospital doctor in the relevant country before being granted generalist status by the national competent authority. Many GPs work independently in continental Europe rather than in British-style group practices and financial outlay at the start can be considerable.

Research

It is possible to plan research abroad either completely or as part of collaborative work. The best way to do this is to contact a head of department in one of the laboratories at home and obtain details of recognized laboratories in the relevant country. Another method is to contact the head of one of the clinical departments in a hospital abroad and ask for contacts in that way.

For clinical research, there are a number of multi-centre trials which are based in various EU and other countries. Contacting either the head of department of a large laboratory or one of the larger drug companies would provide information regarding these. It should be mentioned, though, that these types of trial often do not require additional medical staff and working in this type of research is unlikely to provide an equivalent income to working abroad as a clinical practitioner.

BECOMING REGISTERED AND FINDING EMPLOYMENT

Registration is rather taken for granted by doctors practising within their own country, as it happens almost automatically following qualification. For doctors wishing to work abroad, however, it is necessary to be registered in the destination country in order to practise.

Registration: the practicalities

Each member state has a nominated body or *competent authority* to process applications for registration. Competent authorities operate at regional and national level, depending on country. In the UK, the competent authority is national: the General Medical Council. For doctors who are *citizens* of and who have *completed primary medical training* within an EU member state, it is agreed that the primary medical qualification awarded be recognized in other member states.

There is no centralized registration procedure, so that an incoming doctor is completely at the mercy of the destination country's bureaucracy. However, EC law requires authorities to process applications for qualification *recognition* within 3 months. This is fine, but even once the primary qualification has been recognized, obtaining actual registration can be a complicated and lengthy process. Registration should be applied for well in advance of the appointment start date.

Registration procedures are shown in Figure 3.1.

The European Commission has ruled that authorities may not impose language tests as a condition for registration because this would be a barrier to movement between states. However, a doctor is unlikely to be awarded a post if he or she cannot speak the local language and it is generally agreed that competence in the relevant language is an ethical requirement.

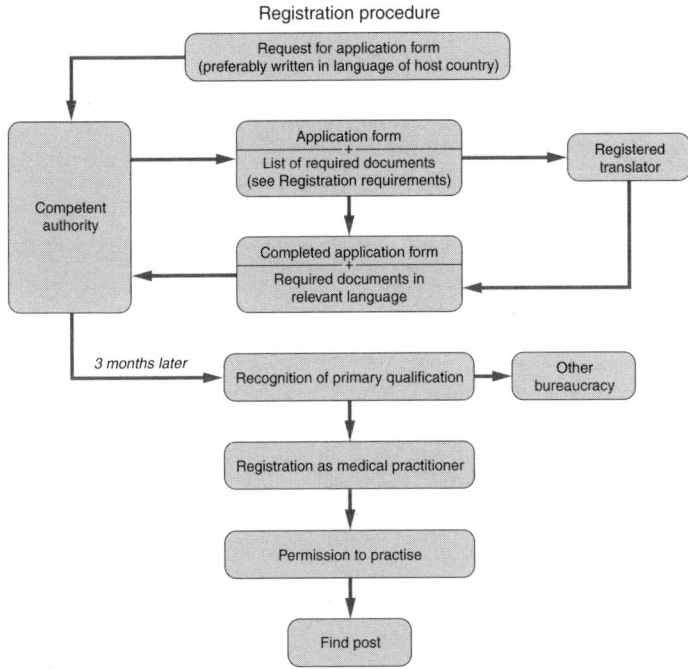

Fig. 3.1 Registration procedure. (NB 'Other bureaucracy' varies from country to country. Belgium probably wins the prize for complexity (see p. 57) with involvement of the National Board of Health, the Medical Commission and the Medical Council. Registration in Belgium can take around 5 months. For any country, applying *at least* 6 months before a post to commence is recommended.

EC legislation suggests that member states establish information centres to distribute details regarding ethics and law to incoming doctors. In Finland and Sweden, a doctor must be aware of the national laws before commencing practice.

Registration requirements vary and the first step is to contact the national competent authority for an application form. When the form is sent, it will be accompanied by a list of the documentation required for that particular member state. The doctor will also be advised whether it is necessary to apply for registration with a *regional* competent authority (as in France) or with the *national* one (as in the UK).

Box 3.1 gives a list of the standard requirements; to save time, the documents can be gathered together while the official application form is awaited.

BOX 3.1
Registration requirements

- Recognized primary qualification which allows full registration as a medical practitioner[1]
- Certificate of full registration[2]
- Certificate of nationality[3]
- Certificate of good character or of good standing[2]
- Curriculum vitae showing medical career

[1] Recognized primary qualifications for each country are listed at the end of each country chapter in Section II.
[2] Issued by the national competent authority; the certificate of good standing must be issued within 3 months of the registration application.
[3] Passport or national identity card.

All the documents in Box 3.1 must be translated into the language of the host country unless otherwise stated. (English is acceptable in some Scandinavian countries.) The translations must be carried out by a recognized official translator. The British Embassy in each member state usually has a list of such people. For doctors coming to the UK, documents can be translated into English at the Berlitz School of Translators (see p. 211 for address). Translation costs vary according to language and length of document but tend to be in the order of around £100 for all the documents listed in Box 3.1.

The cost of registration also varies between countries but this is an unavoidable expense if one plans to practise in the host country. Once registration has been granted, there is also an annual subscription in order to be kept on the national register. Note also that, in some instances, it is necessary to collect or deliver certain documents for registration *in person* and so costs for travel to the host country before beginning employment may be incurred.

Types of registration are listed in Box 3.2.

BOX 3.2
Types of registration

Primary qualification
- Requires that the doctor:
  — Is a citizen of an EU member state
  — Has completed primary training in an EU member state
  — Holds a recognized qualification in accordance with directive 93/16/EC

Specialization
- This is less clear-cut. Moves towards harmonization of specialist training are presently under way. Directive 93/16/EC contains a list of specialties common to all member states and those common to two or more

General practice
- Directive 86/457/EC states that a minimum of 2 years' specific vocational training is required for recognition of generalist status

---

If applying as part of a European exchange scheme, it is possible to begin work without full registration in the host country, as the exchangee has already been recommended by a head of department in a recognized and respected institution. Even so, without the appropriate registration documentation and a registration number, it is not possible to prescribe treatment or even to request investigations, and this is tiresome for all concerned.

Finding a post (see Box 3.3)

Registration is necessary for permission to practise but obtaining it does not guarantee employment. Finding a post depends on language competence and

---

BOX 3.3
Options for finding a post

- Medical journals
- Contacting hospitals
  — Medical staffing/personnel
  — Head of relevant department
- Contacting local health authority
- European schemes in operation
  — European Exchange Scheme
  — Erasmus/Socrates programme

an acquaintance with the proposed host country. Most posts are advertised in the national journals but it is worth enquiring more directly at either one of the main hospitals or the relevant regional health authority to learn of potential vacancies in advance. If looking for employment independently, these are the options and in most of the country chapters, the main medical journals which advertise posts are listed, together with the main teaching hospitals that can be contacted. Where these have not been included, the national medical association or competent authority can provide the relevant information.

It should be mentioned that post availability will vary depending on degree of national unemployment, region (fewer doctors in training are attracted to placements in remote rural areas) and specialty. In some areas, for example, in paediatrics, anaesthetics, psychiatry, oncology and obstetrics and gynaecology posts tend to be relatively undersubscribed, whereas posts in general internal medicine and surgery are usually oversubscribed and competition is fierce.

For doctors with a less than fluent grasp of the host language, working abroad as part of a European exchange scheme may be more practical. This type of scheme, together with the Erasmus/Socrates programme, is described later in this chapter. Both are well organized and provide an ideal opportunity to work abroad, as the host institutions have experience with foreign students and are thus suitably patient and understanding when language skills are less than optimal.

EUROPEAN SCHEMES IN ACTION

Erasmus and Socrates

Erasmus is a European initiative which enables students to study abroad. The scheme has been running for some years but is now part of Socrates.

Socrates is an EC action programme which was launched in 1995 for cooperation in the field of education as a whole — that is, at all levels and in all subjects. It developed from Article 126 of the Treaty on European Union which states that the Community shall 'contribute to the development of quality education'. It is the first European initiative to cover all types and all levels of education, including both students and teaching staff. The programme has been set up drawing from EC programmes launched in specific sectors of education, such as the Erasmus project in higher education and the Lingua programme for European language learning. The Socrates programme includes the 15 EU member states, countries covered by the agreement on the EEA (Iceland, Norway and Liechtenstein), countries in central and eastern Europe, including the Baltic States and the Slovak Republic, and Cyprus.

The European Commission (or more specifically, the Directorate-General XII: Education, Training and Youth) has overall responsibility for implementing Socrates. The Socrates Committee has been set up to assist this implementation and is made up of two members designated by each member state. There are then two sub-committees dealing with each of the fields of higher education and school education. Administration is also decentralized to national level, where it is dealt with by National Agencies designated by the participating countries. The National Agencies have specific responsibilities concerning selection of projects, allocation of grants to students, monitoring and financial management.

Selection of applicants and submission of applications for grants depend on whether the project is centralized and so dealt with by the EC, or decentralized and managed by the National Agencies. The present Commission support for Socrates was to run to the end of 1999. After this there was to be a transitional year but the programme was to continue under the same name. Further information and guidelines for applicants are available from the National Agencies or at the Socrates website (see 'Addresses', below).

Erasmus deals with higher education and this is the section of Socrates that now covers all grades of staff within academic institutions, including medical students, research workers, lecturers and heads of academic departments (professors). The programme organizes exchanges between two institutions for recognized periods of study. The difference between the previous Erasmus programme and the programme incorporated into Socrates is that now both candidates must apply to the respective National Agencies on behalf of their academic institutions rather than as individuals.

Erasmus is divided into two *actions*:

- Action 1 deals with financial support to universities.
- Action 2 deals with mobility grants for students wishing to study in another participating country.

Erasmus candidates must study for a minimum period of 3 months or one academic term, and for a maximum of 1 year. First-year students are not eligible. The partner university and student must agree on the project before the student leaves home. Studies in participating countries must be fully recognized by universities of origin. Host universities do not charge enrolment fees to exchange students and must provide reception arrangements and help with practical problems and accommodation.

The student mobility grants are managed by the National Agencies designated by the participating country and are intended to help cover extra costs incurred by students in their home institution. The grant cannot exceed ECU 5000 per student for a maximum of 12 months abroad or ECU 500 per month for shorter periods. Special provision can be made for students with disabilities, including the award of grants above the maximum.

Further information regarding the Socrates/Erasmus programme should be available from the European Liaison Office of each medical school or from the National Agency. In the UK the National Agency is at the following address:

UK Socrates/Erasmus Council
University of Kent
Canterbury CT2 7PD
Tel: 01227 762 712

It is also possible to visit the Socrates website at http://europa.eu.int/eu/comm/dg22/socrates.htm/ or the Erasmus site at http://www.ukc.ac.uk/ERASMUS/erasmus.

European Exchange Scheme

The European Exchange Scheme has been in operation since 1977. It was the brainchild of Professor Charles van Ypersele de Strihou, who was head of the renal department at a leading academic institution in Brussels. He saw the exchange between different European countries as a means of promoting medical education among junior doctors by exposing them to different health-care systems. The scheme was established with the help of EU funding between leading academic departments in Britain, Belgium and Switzerland. Since the scheme's inception, nearly 200 candidates have taken part, moving between 14 departments of medicine in 8 countries. Centres in the UK, Belgium and the Netherlands have been the most active but exchanges have also taken place in France, Germany, Switzerland, Austria and Portugal.

The heads of department of host centres meet annually to discuss candidates interested in working abroad. The candidates apply in their native countries and so compete against others with similar training backgrounds to obtain a place. As each candidate is effectively an ambassador for his or her country and as host departments are based at academic tertiary centres, prospective applicants must be of reasonable calibre.

Knowledge of the appropriate language is not a prerequisite to be awarded a place but once the post has been confirmed, candidates are obliged to 'brush up' intensively before starting work.

The scheme provides an unparalleled opportunity to work in another member state while bypassing competition for posts with native doctors. It also provides the means for doctors who are proficient but not fluent in a second language to work abroad, as staff in participating departments are prepared for linguistic imperfections and arrange initial work commitments accordingly. Some centres offer a running-in period shadowing a native doctor before assuming full responsibility and there are usually reduced or no on-call duties for the first few weeks.

Participating centres are indicated in each country chapter under the heading 'List of hospitals'. Further information is available from the medical department at these institutions. In the UK, exchange schemes are advertised as part of general medical rotations in the *BMJ* but one-off, purely European appointments are possible if planned in advance. The placements tend to be for 6 months to 1 year and are arranged mainly at SHO level, but negotiation has been possible. In theory, if two heads of department can get together, each with a well-motivated candidate, an exchange can be developed to best fit both parties, provided it is within EU guidelines.

The exchange scheme is well organized and, because it operates between teaching hospitals of high standard, is highly beneficial to overall medical training.

COST

A change in post frequently incurs changes in other areas, be it with respect to travel arrangements, salary differences or simple daily routine. Clearly, starting a post in another country will bring about changes on a rather larger scale and these have their price.

The financial aspects of moving and working abroad are not inconsiderable and ought to be addressed well in advance. Financial outlay occurs even before taking up the new post and a 'European experience' is not advised for those badly in the red.

In the world of commerce and enterprise, there is usually some form of relocation allowance for employees of large companies. This is seldom the case in medicine. Doctors in training tend to be transitory beings and hospital trusts do not 'owe' them more than their present employment. Host countries are not short of staff and it is not particularly in their interest to have an influx of foreigners. It is worth assuming, therefore, that only limited financial help (if any) will be provided from one's current place of work.

The points listed in Box 3.4 are discussed below.

How to go about planning the move abroad will depend on how long one intends to stay.

Leaving home

For those in rented property, a move elsewhere is relatively simple. For home owners, the choice is between selling or letting. If selling is out, continuing

> **BOX 3.4**
> **The cost of moving abroad: a checklist**
>
> **Transfer costs**
> - Transport to and from host country
> - Relocation of belongings
> - Forwarding mail
>
> **Getting started**
> - Language courses
> - Translation of documents required for registration
> - Travel to competent authority to deliver/collect documents
> - Visit to future place of employment
> - Registration fee + annual subscription to local competent authority
>
> **Accommodation**
> - Rent +/− bills/insurance
> - Management of property at home while away
>
> **Salary**
> - Salary differences between countries
> - ? On-call work paid
> - Exchange rates if paid in local currency
>
> **Family**
> - Schooling / crèche
>
> **General**
> - NHS pension plan contributions while away
> - Insurance (see Box 3.5)
>
> **Non-financial**
> - General upheaval
> - Career structure

payment of the mortgage, if applicable, needs to be arranged. Letting is an additional source of income but having someone trustworthy on site is recommended, as matters such as rent-chasing and property upkeep are difficult to manage from afar.

Moving belongings

Again, this depends on how long the period abroad is to be. If the post is for the short to medium term, moving just one's essential belongings is more sensible, given that the whole lot will only have to be brought back again at the end. Keeping things to a minimum saves on transport costs but putting belongings into storage is another outlay.

If professional help is required, numerous removal companies exist for the transfer of goods within Europe on a company or individual basis. For those travelling light, without furniture, they are probably not necessary, but perhaps should be borne in mind for the return journey. The alternative is to hire a van.

Change of address

The advice here is to plan ahead and to contact everyone imaginable. The checklist in Box 3.5 is provided as a guide. The local post office in Britain will

---

BOX 3.5
Planning a move abroad: a checklist

(Important points are in italic type)
Employment
- Contract: terms and conditions
- ? Salary: ? *payment for on-call work*
- If exchange, *which country pays salary?*
- ? *Recognized for overall training requirements*
- *Registration with country's competent authority*

Accommodation
- At home: mortgage/letting/selling
- Abroad: price — ? inclusive of bills / *insurance* / furnished / unfurnished

Insurance (ensure cover is provided abroad as well as at home)
- Health
- Belongings
- Accommodation at home and abroad
- Car
- *Medical indemnity*
- *Critical illness cover and personal injury plan*

Car
- Driving licence
- Vehicle registration (road taxation)
- Insurance

Notification of change of address
- Friends and relations
- Electricity, gas, water, telephone
- Council tax
- Bank, stocks and shares dividends
- Insurance
- Journals

Other
- Transport of belongings
- Schooling for children / crèche facilities

forward mail for a period of 3, 6 or 12 months, for a cost of £13 upwards, depending on the period the service is to cover and the destination. One week's notice is required.

Rent

Assuming arrangements at home have been settled, accommodation abroad is the next issue to address. Rent levels will vary from country to country and will also depend on the location within a given town. In general, accommodation categories can be divided into furnished and unfurnished. The costs of the former are not always superior to those of the latter. In addition, care should be taken with unfurnished property, as often the responsibility of the tenant with respect to property upkeep is far greater. Beware of the small print regarding legal matters and insurance (of both contents and building — see below).

Home insurance

If household contents are already insured, it is important to ascertain whether this policy covers the transport of belongings and whether the goods will still be insured at their destination, either in storage or during the placement abroad.

Insurance costs for house contents aside, note that it is vital to establish who takes responsibility for insurance of the *building*. This varies from country to country and from landlord to landlord, but a tenant must be covered in case of damage to property, even in the case of natural disasters.

Finding accommodation abroad

Finding accommodation can cause problems; having somewhere to go on arrival is desirable but not if it involves paying rent for weeks in advance. Employing only letting agencies that have been recommended cannot be advised strongly enough. Often, the hospital secretaries will have some helpful advice. The one perk of working in a teaching hospital is that there is usually an academic centre nearby which has a list of accommodation for medical students. Student flats are a possibility, if only for the short term, and would provide a base from which to seek something more suitable. Nurses' residences provide a similar solution.

Salary changes

Beware! Salaries vary between countries for a given doctor grade. Jobs with fewer hours per week or with unpaid on-call duty pay less and this can add up, given all the other costs involved in relocating. The importance of anticipating outgoing costs with respect to future salary cannot be overemphasized.

For exchange posts, it is necessary to establish which health authority pays the salary. The other point to consider for all posts is whether or not the salary is affected by exchange rate. That is, is the salary paid in one's native currency and converted to local currency or is it converted to local currency equivalent at the start and then maintained at that level for the duration of the time abroad?

These points must be clarified before starting, but again, beware. Contracts are generally written in the local language and in your first few weeks away certain financial or legal subtleties may be lost on you. There is no way of being refunded later if errors are made at the start. (Exchange scheme organizers have argued in the past, perhaps with just cause, that if the reverse occurred and doctors were paid above their usual salary, they would be unlikely to volunteer to return the difference.)

Language improvement

Starting any job takes some getting used to and fretting about syntax inadequacies simply adds to general anxiety. For those not fluent in the host country's language, some brushing-up is recommended before starting. This provides another expense.

Costs for language improvement range from investing in a decent dictionary or grammar guide to taking a one-to-one language course. Language courses vary in expense depending on class size and on whether they take place at home or in the native country. Evening classes at home can provide a basis, but for more rapid learning a crash course in the native country, although more expensive, is probably more efficient.

Caledonia Languages is a UK-based firm which has been running since 1994. Its advantage is that it deals only with language schools that are known to it and that have a good track record. It is possible to arrange language courses with impressive convenience in terms of level of teaching, duration of course and time of year. The course fee includes accommodation either with a native family or in a self-catering establishment close to the language school. The people involved bend over backwards to try to accommodate each customer's demands, while giving frank advice about what is and is not possible. This firm has well-established contacts for courses in French, German, Spanish, Italian, Portuguese, Greek, Dutch and English, all based in the relevant countries. Special requests, notably for courses concentrating on medical terminology, can be arranged. It would be worth enquiring about Scandinavian languages; although no course has as yet been set up, the firm may be able to give advice on how to proceed. For further information contact:

Kath Bateman, Proprietor
Caledonia Languages Abroad
The Clockhouse
Bonnington Mill
72 Newhaven Road
Edinburgh EH6 5QG
Tel: 0131 621 7721/2
Fax: 0131 621 7723
e-mail: info@caledonialanguages.co.uk
http://www.caledonialanguages.co.uk

Registration

As discussed earlier, a doctor cannot practise without registration with the competent authority of the host member state. The process of registration has been described and is covered in detail in each specific country chapter. As well as registration fees and annual subscriptions, other expenses include payment for document translation and travel costs when certain documents need to be collected or delivered in person. While in the host country to deal with registration, however, one can always make the most of the trip and visit the future place of employment, thereby saving money in the long run.

General finance

Other aspects to be considered include:

- income protection plans (IPPs)
- critical illness cover (CIC)
- taxation
- pension plans.

For IPP and CIC policies, one should ensure before leaving that cover is provided for work in the new host country. The same applies for medical indemnity (see below).

A person who has lived in another member state for less than 3 years retains the title of 'expatriate' and is therefore entitled to a reduction in tax payments. Tax is none the less deducted from hospital salaries and contributions towards local pension funds or health insurance cannot be claimed back.

While one is working outside the NHS, there is no upkeep of the NHS pension scheme. This issue should be addressed in advance either so that payment can continue in instalments or a lump sum on return, or else so that one can accept the fact that the dividends at retirement will suffer.

Under EU regulations, workers based in two or more EU countries should be able to combine the state pension contributions paid in each country in order to qualify for a pension. For more information, contact the Overseas Branch of the DSS at the following address:

Department of Social Security
Overseas Branch
Newcastle upon Tyne NE98 1YX

For all insurance policies (household and contents, travel, health, car, life assurance, medical indemnity), make sure cover extends to the place and conditions of work abroad. Information on car insurance and other vehicle regulations is available free from the local vehicle registration office or from the Driver and Vehicle Licensing Centre in Swansea.

Driving

Petrol and other running costs vary between countries. Driving is particularly expensive in Denmark, and in Sweden cars are required to pass a strict roadworthiness test.

Since January 1983 driving licences obtained in an EU country have been valid for other member states so it is not necessary for EU nationals to resit driving tests locally.

A vehicle taken abroad should be licensed either with the local vehicle registration office or with the registration office at home. (In the UK this is the Driver and Vehicle Licensing Centre.)

Family considerations

Accommodation is a bigger issue if there is more than one person to consider, and proximity to schools may also be required. In most EU countries, government schools exist where no fees are necessary. Many large towns now have international schools or schools where English is spoken. These are sparse in smaller towns and rural areas.

Non-financial costs

Moving abroad is a hassle. It involves a lot of organization, largely in advance, often when one is already working in a demanding job with difficult hours and time is limited for making big plans. Motivation is vital but being well prepared will help plans go more smoothly. Anticipated obstacles are easier to deal with than bolts from the blue.

Moving abroad can also be unsettling, as it means leaving behind family and friends and a daily routine. This is not always a bad thing, but for those with a spouse and children the upheaval is multiplied. It is important to make sure that an interesting career experience is not to the detriment of a child's education; working in a country whose culture is compatible with general family harmony is as important as finding a suitable school.

Career

Until recently, mention of a sabbatical abroad on the curriculum vitae was either overlooked completely or regarded in a negative light. This is now changing and training supervisors actually encourage a 'European experience' during the training period. For the moment, however, the Royal College of Physicians is unwilling to promise acknowledgement of a post abroad as eligible to count towards overall training, although the word 'probably' is used. This is largely owing to the differing quality of medical training in the EU. As mentioned in Chapter 2, posts will be credited more highly in some countries than in others.

Depending on how one goes about it, working abroad can be a risk with respect to overall career plans but this is becoming less and less the case. It is always advisable to discuss any potential posts abroad with a clinical tutor and to write directly to the General Professional Training department at the Royal College of Physicians. If acknowledgement is given for any appointment abroad, this must be obtained *in writing*.

As mentioned throughout this book, working in another country is a fascinating experience to be recommended to anyone prepared to wander off more conventional training paths. It is useful for medical training as a whole to work with other indigenous populations and their diseases, in different health-care systems. It is refreshing to experience variety in this way and if the risk is achieving consultancy at 37 instead of 36, it is probably worth the gamble.

SECTION 2

Country chapters

Austria

Joined EU: 1995
Area: 84 000 km²
Population (1998): 8.13 million
Population density: 97 persons / km²
Language: German
Currency: Schilling
Religion: Roman Catholic (78%)
Government: Federal republic
GDP per head (1994): 18 829 US$
Health expenditure as % of GDP (1995): 7.9%
Infant mortality rate (1998): 5.16 deaths per 1000 live births
Average life expectancy at birth (1998): 74.1 (men); 80.7 (women); total 77.3 years
Unemployment (1995): 7.1%
Doctors per 10 000 population (1995): 26.6
Beds per 10 000 population (1995): 9.3

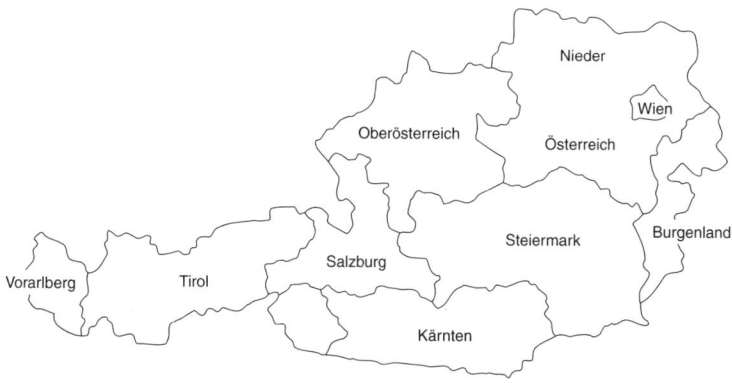

Fig. 4.1 Map of Austria.

BACKGROUND

Austria was re-established as an independent state in 1955 and is now a presidential federal republic with a two-house national assembly. Situated on the eastern edge of the EU, Austria has close relations with the emerging nations of eastern Europe, particularly Hungary. The country is divided into semi-autonomous regions called Länder.

Almost half the country is covered by forest and the western Tyrol region is mountainous. The majority of the population and most of the main towns, including the capital city, Vienna, are in the east.

Taxation and social security payments are high, as is the cost of living.

Education is free and compulsory from 6–15 years.

LANGUAGE

German is the national language of Austria (see Chapter 9).

ORGANIZATION OF THE HEALTH SYSTEM

The present health-care system in Austria dates from 1956.

Health insurance

Around 99% of the population has some form of social insurance and over one-third has complementary private insurance. The social insurance schemes differ according to the cover provided (health care, accident and / or pensions) and type of employment (self-employed, civil servants, those in agriculture and forestry, unemployed). The premiums which finance the scheme are fixed by law and have an upper limit. They are income-related, so are higher for certain groups such as farmers and the self-employed. For those not self-employed, 50% of insurance contributions come from the employee and 50% from the employer.

The schemes are primarily the responsibility of the Ministry of Social Affairs, rather than the Ministry of Health, and cover not only the insured person but also his or her dependants. Although more than half of health-care funding comes from insurance (social or private), there are smaller contributions from taxations and co-payments. The latter apply to simple (non-emergency) hospital care, drugs and some dental care.

Finance

Hospitals are funded by the insurance contributions, with additional income from the State. Psychiatric hospitals are subsidized to a large extent by the government. Plans for changing the hospital finance system are currently being introduced.

Hospital types

Hospitals can be categorized as public or state-run, and private. Public-sector physicians are state employees and receive a salary. Doctors working with a social insurance company contract are paid on a fee-for-service basis (*Vertragärtze*).

Access to specialist care

Patients who have social insurance must carry evidence of registration with an insurance scheme (*Krankenkassenscheck*) when receiving medical care in order to be reimbursed later on. There are over 20 social insurance bodies, organized according to Länder. They have considerable autonomy and own public hospitals which are not owned expressly by the government.

Austria does not run a gatekeeper system, so that patients have freedom to consult any specialist they choose. Provided they carry the *Krankenkassenscheck*, they are reimbursed according to the treatment they receive. Co-payments are charged for some services, as described above.

TRAINING AND TYPES OF POST

Entry to university is available to anyone who has completed secondary education. A *numerus clausus* has been introduced from the first year so that student numbers are much reduced by the time clinical studies begin.

Training includes a period as an intern before full registration is awarded.

Specialist recognition is subject to competent authority approval. Once training requirements have been met, the specialist diploma (*Facharztdiplom*) is awarded.

REGISTRATION

Although there is no formal language testing procedure, a reasonable grasp of German is required before work in Austria can be considered, as all the necessary paperwork sent out by the competent authority is in German.

To obtain registration, an application form is required from the national competent authority, the *Österreichische Ärztekammer* (see 'Addresses', below). This body issues information regarding registration requirements according to applicant nationality and a list of the registration bodies (*Landesärztekammer*) for each province. Registration is dealt with at provincial level according to where employment is to be based.

The necessary documents (which include the primary diploma, certificate of registration with the native competent authority, certificate of nationality and certificate of good standing) must be translated into German by a recognized translator and sent to the appropriate provincial competent authority, together with two passport-sized photographs and a registration fee (around 560 Austrian Schillings). Once registration has been approved, training hospital registration (*Ausbildungsstattenverzeichnis*) is awarded and the doctor is eligible to apply for a post.

FINDING A POST

The Austrian and Vienna Medical Association is at the same address as the national competent authority and provides advice on finding employment. All the information is in German but some English is spoken by people answering the telephones. The three university hospitals in Austria are listed below. They can be contacted directly for details regarding short-term employment.

LIST OF HOSPITALS

Kliniken d Universität
Abteilung für Notfallmedizin
Währinger Gürtel 18–20
A-1090 Wien
Tel: 00 43 (0) 1 402 5777

Allgemeines Krankenhaus der Stadt Wien
Universitätsklinik für Innere Medezin III
Währinger Gürtel 18–20
A-1090 Wien
Tel: 00 43 (0) 1 40400 4390
Fax: 00 43 (0) 1 40400 4392

Exchange scheme

Kliniken Allg öfentl Landeskrankenhaus (Universitätskliniken)
Anichst 35
A-6020 Innsbruck
Tel: 00 43 (0) 512 504 2000
Fax: 00 43 (0) 512 504 2011
Tel: 00 43 (0) 512 504 3255 ⎫ Internal medicine
Fax: 00 43 (0) 512 504 3391 ⎭

Landeskrankenhaus — Universitätskliniken Graz
Auenbruggerplatz 1
A-8036 Graz
Tel: 00 43 (0) 316 385 2242
Fax: 00 43 (0) 316 385 3422

ADDRESSES

Competent authority *Vienna*
Österreichische Ärztekammer
Weihburggasse 10–12
1010 Wien
Tel: 00 43 (0) 1 5150 1253
Fax: 00 43 (0) 1 5150 1410

Addresses of the Landesärztekammer for each Austrian province are as follows:

Salzburg
Bergstrasse 14
5024 Salzburg
Tel: 00 43 (0) 732 778371–0

Oberösterreich
Dinghoferstrasse 4
4010 Linz
Tel: 00 43 (0) 732 778371–0

Niederösterreich
Wipplingerstrasse 2
1010 Wien
Tel: 00 43 (0) 222 5333611–0

Burgenland
Permayerstrasse 3
7000 Eisenstadt
Tel: 00 43 (0) 2682 625 21

Steiermark
Kaiserfeldgasse 29
8011 Graz
Tel: 00 43 (0) 316 8044–0

Kärnten
St Veiterstrasse 34
9020 Klagenfurt
Tel: 00 43 (0) 463 58 56–0

Tirol
Anichstrasse 7/IV
6010 Innsbruck
Tel: 00 43 (0) 512 52058

Vorarlberg
Schulgasse 17
6850 Dornbirn
Tel: 00 43 (0) 5572 21900–0

Wien Vienna
Weihburggasse 10–12
1010 Wien
Tel: 00 43 (0) 222 51501–0

REGISTRABLE QUALIFICATIONS FOR AUSTRIAN DOCTORS GOING ABROAD

The registrable qualification granted in Austria is the *Doktor der gesamten Heilkunde* (diploma of doctor of medicine), awarded by a university faculty of medicine, and the *Diplom über die spezialiste Ausbildung in der Algemeinmedizin* (diploma of specialist training in general medicine), or *Facharztdiplom* (diploma of specialist doctor), issued by the competent authority.

The *Bescheinigung über die Absolvierung der Tätigkeit Arzt im Praktikum* (certificate of practical training), supposedly also awarded by the competent authority and asked for by some competent authorities for registration (notably France), has in fact never existed and the basic diploma is sufficient.

There are twelve universities in Austria, of which three have a faculty of medicine. They award the following qualifications:

- Universität Innsbruck: *MD Innsbruck*
- Universität Wien: *MD Wien*
- Universität Graz: *MD Graz*.

Further information for medical students is available from:

Austrian Academic Exchange Service (ÖAD)
Zentrale Geschäftsstelle
Universität Wien
1/Stiege 9
A-1010 Wien
Tel: 00 43 (0) 1 426742

A booklet entitled, 'Information for foreign students intending to study at an Austrian institution of higher learning' is available from this address.

Belgium

Joined EU: 1957
Area: 30 500 km^2
Population (1998): 10.18 million
Population density: 334 persons / km^2
Languages: Dutch (57%); French (32%); bilingual Dutch/French (9%); German (0.7%)
Currency: Belgian franc
Religion: Roman Catholic (75%)
Government: Federal parliamentary democracy under constitutional monarchy
GDP per head (1994): 18 800 US$
Social security expenditure as % of GDP (1993): 26.3%
Health expenditure as % of GDP (1995): 8.0%
Infant mortality rate (1998): 6.27 deaths per 1000 live births
Average life expectancy at birth (1998): 74.1 (men); 80.7 (women); total 77.4 years
Unemployment (1997): 12.8%
Doctors per 10 000 population (1994): 37.4
Beds per 10 000 population (1994): 7.6

BACKGROUND

Belgium, famous for Tintin, chocolates, chips and mayonnaise, is a growing destination for British doctors wishing to work abroad. Although at first sight the country appears small and slightly reclusive, it is in fact a hive of high-quality medical activity. As mentioned in the European Exchange Scheme section (see p. 32), one of the founders of this scheme was based at a large Brussels teaching hospital and Belgium has played host to the majority of exchangees.

Belgium is a constitutional and hereditary monarchy. The country can be

GUIDE TO WORKING IN EUROPE FOR DOCTORS

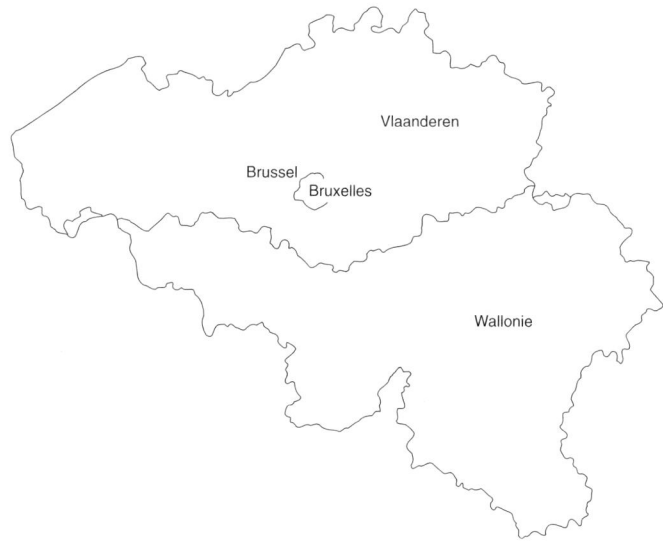

Fig. 5.1 Map of Belgium.

divided geographically into the coastal plain, central plateau and Ardennes highlands; or politically/culturally into the three regions of Flanders, Brussels and Wallonia. Flemish is spoken in Flanders and French in Wallonia. In Brussels, which is an enclave of Flanders, the official language is French, and in the eastern *cantons* of Belgium, German is spoken. Belgium is divided into 10 provinces and nearly 600 *communes* (administrative districts).

The historical and present-day political complexity of Belgium belies its size. Until the Second World War, French-speaking Wallonia, with its coal and steel industries, was the economic stronghold of Belgium. In the 1950s, light industries began to flourish in the north of the country and Flanders became increasingly prosperous. The Flems and Walloons have never really got on, and in the post-war period friction continued to grow. The Flems began to consider Wallonia an economic drain and the Walloons felt unjustly treated. In 1971, Belgium began to undergo constitutional change and turned towards a federal monarchy, giving political recognition to the different language communities. A new constitution of elected assemblies and governments representing each linguistic group was created. The process was completed in May 1993.

Differences continue, however, and there are concerns that further devolution is likely. Up to now, health care has remained uniform throughout Belgium in spite of the different governments. However, with the Flemish community being generally wealthier with fewer unemployed and less morbidity, some consider that the health insurance costs for this group could be reduced and the health-care system could be made more efficient if the two communities were separated. Belgium thus faces total division of its health care between the Flemish- and French-speaking communities. Moves towards this split, if agreed, would begin in 1999.

Anyone planning to stay in Belgium must register at the local town hall (*la commune*) within 8 days of arrival. The officials there notify the police and issue a provisional identity card. It is a legal requirement for residents to carry a certificate of identity, either an identity card or a passport, at all times.

Cars must be registered either in Belgium or in one's native country. Drivers should beware of the *priorité à droite* rule, whereby all cars coming from the right must be given right of way. This extends to cars turning on to a major thoroughfare and includes some major roundabouts, although anticipating which drivers adhere to these rules is rather left to chance.

Taxes are considerable (up to 40% of gross salary) and include income tax, municipal tax and a crisis contribution surcharge. In theory, expatriates not permanently resident in Belgium are entitled to tax concessions. In practice, it is difficult to find anyone to confirm this.

Education is free and compulsory from 6–18 years.

Perhaps with the capital city being the 'capital of Europe' and consequently having a higher-than-average quota of civil servants, there is a lot of form-filling in Belgium and bureaucracy abounds with ever-increasing complexity. It is useful to bear this in mind while undertaking administrative procedures.

On the more positive side, one of the attractions of Brussels is the diverse mix of nationalities, particularly around the EU headquarters. Incoming professionals find they can integrate relatively quickly as people in Brussels are used to socializing with all nationalities. As the country has two official languages, people who have a grasp of either French or Dutch can apply for work in Belgium. This then opens up opportunities for placements in France or the Netherlands.

LANGUAGE

Flemish is spoken in the northern half of the country by around 5.5 million people (slightly more than half the population). It is in fact the same language as Dutch but cultural and religious distinctions over the centuries have led to the use of separate terms for the same language. Otherwise there are differences in accent. Amongst these is the soft pronunciation of the letter *g*; in Flemish, it is more of a breathy *h* sound than the harsher *ch* (as in Scottish *loch*) sound of Dutch.

French and German are also spoken (see Chapters 8 and 9).

ORGANIZATION OF THE HEALTH SYSTEM

Health-care responsibility is shared on a national level by the Ministry of Public Health and the Dutch-, French- and German-speaking Community Ministries of Health. The former is in charge of social services and hospital financing, while the latter deal with hospital accreditation procedures and preventative medicine.

The 10 provincial communities deal with social assistance for people on low incomes. They are also in charge of the organization of emergency services, although the financing of these services is the government's responsibility. The provincial medical councils are responsible for checking the authenticity of non-Belgian doctors' qualifications and for issuing registration numbers (the INAMI number — see below).

Health insurance

Health care in Belgium is based on a system of compulsory health insurance whereby everyone has to belong to a sickness insurance fund (*une mutuelle*). Insurance payments, which are linked to degree of patient dependency, are distributed by the National Institute of Sickness and Invalidity Insurance to six recognized insurance funds. The health insurance scheme covers almost the whole population and is supported by government subsidies, which account for over one-third of total funding. The government has a role in regulating the system but providers of health care have a considerable degree of independence.

Medical fees paid by patients are reimbursed by insurance funds according to social status and type of care received. This is around 75% normally, but can be up to 100% for the elderly and unemployed.

Treatment charges are reimbursed according to treatment category. All products are itemized, from prescribed drugs and intravenous fluids including blood products to baby milk. Drugs are classified into four categories to determine the level of reimbursement — for example, 'life-savers' are reimbursed at 100%. A negotiated list of prescription drugs has been compiled by the Ministry of Public Health to be sold under special regulations and classifications at a legally fixed price. For example, certain peptic ulcer treatments, notably proton pump inhibitors, are reimbursed only if the medical prescription is accompanied by the gastroscopy report stating that an ulcer is present — in other words, no gastroscopy, no reimbursement. It is perhaps because of this that patients in Belgium seem more ready to undergo invasive procedures than those in other European countries. The general level of medical knowledge amongst lay people is also comparatively high, perhaps because patients need this information to ascertain whether their outgoing costs for treatment are eligible for reimbursement.

Finance

For hospital care, up to 60% of capital expenditure is funded by central government. An annual budget is allocated to each hospital by the Ministry of Public Health based on daily unit cost multiplied by the quota of patient days. The remainder of hospital funds is recovered through hospital charges (hotel costs, medical fees and prescription charges) and raised through bank loans.

Medical fees for patients are based on a national schedule of medical services, negotiated between health insurance bodies 'and the national association of doctors. In the hospital setting, most doctors are salaried and patient fees go towards general hospital income. Doctors in private practice, both within and outside hospitals, operate on a fee-for-service basis. The fees are shared with the clinics whose facilities are used.

Hospital types

Almost all Belgian hospitals are non-profit-making private (presently accounting for two-thirds of hospital beds) or public organizations. For hospital employees, the difference between the two is that in private hospitals, which were originally founded by religious orders and charitable organizations, the personnel have a *contract of work* with their employer, whereas in public hospitals, which were established by municipal councils, the personnel are *government employees*. Another difference is that public hospitals are controlled by central or local government, whereas private hospitals have greater autonomy, being responsible for their own financial administration and management.

Hospitals can also be divided according to degree of specialization and into provincial (district general) and university hospitals. There are no single-specialty hospitals in Belgium, apart from those dealing with psychiatric or care of the elderly services. Recently, non-hospital care for elderly/chronically ill patients has been promoted in an effort to control hospital growth. In psychiatric care, the number of long-stay beds has been reduced, the quality of acute care has improved and more places have been created in sheltered housing.

Access to specialist care

Patients have the right to consult any physician of their choice as often as they please. Outpatient consultations are paid up-front by the patient. He or she then receives reimbursement from the *mutuelle* (insurance fund). For inpatient care, the *mutuelle* pays the hospital directly by third-party payment.

As there is no gatekeeper system, there is no clear distinction between the roles of GPs and of specialists, and in some cases both provide primary care. This increases the level of choice but means that the system lacks lines of referral. It also requires a certain degree of medical knowledge on the part of the patient and people may self-refer inappropriately to certain specialists, simply because they have been recommended.

In spite of such freedom of choice, waiting lists are uncommon but do exist for highly specialized procedures such as renal dialysis, which are unequally distributed throughout the country. In any case, proposals for a gatekeeper system continue to be strongly opposed by the medical profession. In fact, the only incidence of strikes amongst doctors in Belgium was in 1979, in protest against this and against the establishment of a national health service.

TRAINING AND TYPES OF POST

The oldest university with a medical faculty dates from the Middle Ages, being founded under religious auspices in 1425 in Leuven (Louvain). As part of national reforms in 1970, the university was divided into independent French- and Flemish-speaking institutions with some degree of acrimony. The Free University of Brussels, which was established in 1834, also became two independent French and Flemish institutions in 1970. The other universities with faculties of medicine are listed at the end of this chapter, under 'Registrable qualifications for Belgian doctors going abroad'.

Access to medical studies is available to anyone who has successfully completed 18+ education. Successful school-leavers can thus begin a 3-year course in general medical science without specific grades or interview, provided they can afford their own upkeep. At the end of the 3 years, successful candidates (around 20% of the initial intake) can then start the *doctorat* course, as a *stagiaire* (trainee). Students failing the examination at the end of the third year are left with no place in medical school and no degree or other recognition of the preceding years of study.

The period as a *stagiaire* lasts for 4 years: 2 years pre-clinical, followed by 2 years on the wards. The *stagiaires* of the third and fourth *doctorat* years are required to clerk the patients and perform various tasks necessary for the smooth running of the medical team, which include asking other teams for specialist opinions and searching for radiographs. They work similar hours to their superiors but do not receive a salary. The standard of medical knowledge is slightly higher than that of their British counterparts but their clinical interpretation is less strong. Although their function is similar to a PRHO or SHO, they are not authorized to prescribe medication.

Towards the end of the fourth and final year, a student may sit a *concours* (examination) in one of the disciplines (medicine, surgery, gynaecology, etc.)

or else practise as a generalist (*médecin traitant*) in the community. Those who are successful in the *concours*, which is highly competitive and also dependent on grades from in-course assessment, commence the period as *assistant(e)* in the chosen speciality. The period of *assistant* training lasts for 5–6 years, depending on specialty. The first 2–3 years of training are based in general internal medicine, after which time training in a specialty begins. There are no post-graduate examinations in order to pass from 'junior' to 'senior' grade, although doctors in training are required to keep a logbook. At the end of the 5–6 years, the *assistant* is eligible for a post at *résident(e)* grade and so on, as listed in Table 5.1.

Table 5.1 Equivalent grades between Belgium and the UK

Belgium	UK
Academic centres and teaching hospitals	
Stagiaire	
Years 1–2	Pre-clinical medical student
Year 3	Final-year medical student
Year 4	Pre-registration house officer
Assistant(e)	
Years 1–3	Senior house officer
Years 4–5/6	Registrar
Résident(e)	Senior registrar/Specialist registrar in final 1–2 years
Chef de clinique	Junior consultant
Chef de clinique associé(e)	Consultant
Chef de service	Senior consultant
Chef de départment	Head of department
Periphery (district hospitals)	
Médecin permanent	(Non-academic) junior consultant
Chef de service	Senior consultant

PRACTICAL POINTS

Terms and conditions

Assistants generally work from 8.30am to 6.30pm, with on-call commitments varying according to specialty and institution. Hours worked on call are not paid and so a doctor working a 1 in 5 rota will earn the same as one on a 1 in 15. The salary is significantly lower than in the UK (up to 60% less) and taxation is heavy, and so it is important to establish which country is paying the salary of those taking part in a European exchange. On the other hand, the cost of living in Belgium is marginally lower than in France or the UK. Consumables are cheaper, although electrical goods are usually more expensive.

Although on-call duty is unpaid, importance is attached to the availability of food throughout the out-of-hours period. This may not completely make up for the drop in salary for everyone but food in Belgium is pretty good.

Nursing

In teaching hospitals, the standard of nursing is high. Staff have a good knowledge of therapeutics and more freedom with regard to prescribing while awaiting the doctor's signature than in some other EU member states. Nurses also perform such duties as phlebotomy, venous cannulation, intravenous drug administration and even blood gas measurement, both in casualty and on the wards.

Specialization

In teaching hospitals, specialization is taken very seriously. Renal physicians deal with hyponatraemia, respiratory physicians are called to tap pleural effusions, neurologists perform lumbar punctures, anaesthetists insert central lines and so on. Even the crash team (ARCA: Arrêt cardiaque) is specialized, providing 24-hour cover by ITU staff, rather than the familiar bleep-carrying medical registrar on call.

Paperwork

Sadly, the medical profession is not exempt from the country's bureaucracy. Substantial paperwork is generated by the insurance-based health system in the form of certificates of hospital admission and of justification for certain investigations and treatments. Without these, patients do not receive reimbursement and hospital clinics do not get paid. Such form-filling is the duty of the hospital (prescribing) doctor and cannot be simply handed over to the patient's general practitioner.

SAMU

An interesting francophone development is the SAMU (Service d'aide médicale urgente), which also exists in France. Ambulance services in Belgium are private concerns. Ambulance drivers drive ambulances and have no paramedical skills. The principle of the SAMU is that, instead of patients in the community being met by a team of paramedics and brought to hospital, medical staff are taken to the scene and perform the necessary treatment on site. Once the patient is stabilized, he or she is fast-tracked to the nearest centre, depending on situation. In this way, for example, a patient with chest pain can be seen in his or her kitchen at home, obtain an ECG tracing and be treated before being taken straight to the nearest CCU, perhaps even bypassing casualty. Already, a significant impact on morbidity and mortality figures has been made. I mention SAMU particularly because *assistants* on call in casualty can unwittingly be dragged out in an emergency if the regular team is otherwise engaged.

REGISTRATION

Registration is necessary in order to obtain an INAMI (Institut National d'Assurance Maladie-Invalidité) number. This must be stamped on all official documents related to patient care and is necessary for prescribing treatment and for ordering investigations. Starting a job without registration is feasible for doctors working as part of a European exchange but causes problems. Without a stamp with one's name and number one cannot sign even blood request forms, let alone prescribe treatment.

The process of registration in Belgium is a song and dance, to say the least, and involves several authorities (see Box 5.1). The whole procedure can take up to 6 months, in spite of the official EU 3-month time limit for approval of a member state citizen's medical qualifications, and is a disheartening experience for the uninitiated.

BOX 5.1
The principal Belgian authorities involved in registration

- Association of Doctors (Ordre des Médecins)
- Ministry of Health (Ministère de la Santé Publique)
- Provincial Medical Commission (Commission Médicale Provinciale)*
- Provincial Medical Council (Conseil Provincial de l'Ordre de Médecins)
- National Institute of Sickness and Invalidity Insurance (INAMI)

*Although registration takes place in the province where the place of employment is located, it is no longer necessary to re-register when moving to another province.

The Ordre des Médecins is the competent authority, to which the following documents must be submitted (see Fig. 5.2):

- certified copy of the primary qualification, which gives entitlement to registration as a fully registered medical practitioner
- certificate of full registration issued by the doctor's native competent authority
- certificate of nationality (member state of the EEC) (passport)

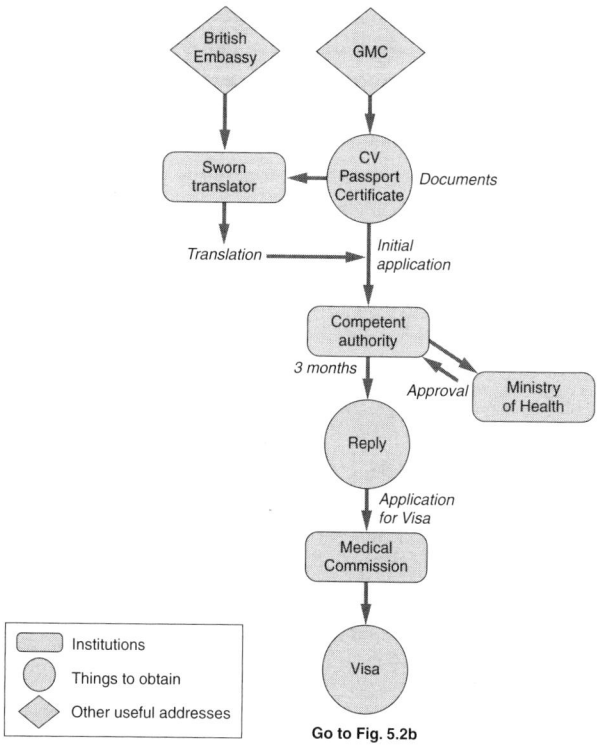

Fig. 5.2a The process of registration in Belgium.

- proof of good character or good repute[1]
- certificate of good standing issued by the doctor's native competent authority (Article 12 of Directive No 93/16/EC)[2]
- curriculum vitae describing one's medical career.

[1]This is theoretically available from the British Embassy but, in practice, such a document is no longer issued and in fact is not actually needed for registration.
[2]For British doctors this is available from the GMC at a cost of £40 for three certificates which are valid for a period of 3 months.

These documents must be sent both in the original (sending a photocopy of the originals is recommended, as often one never sees the papers again) and translated by a *sworn translator*. A list of such translators is available from the British Embassy in Brussels. Translation of documents costs around £150. As charges are made according to length of document, it is worth condensing any unnecessary information. The curriculum vitae, for example, should

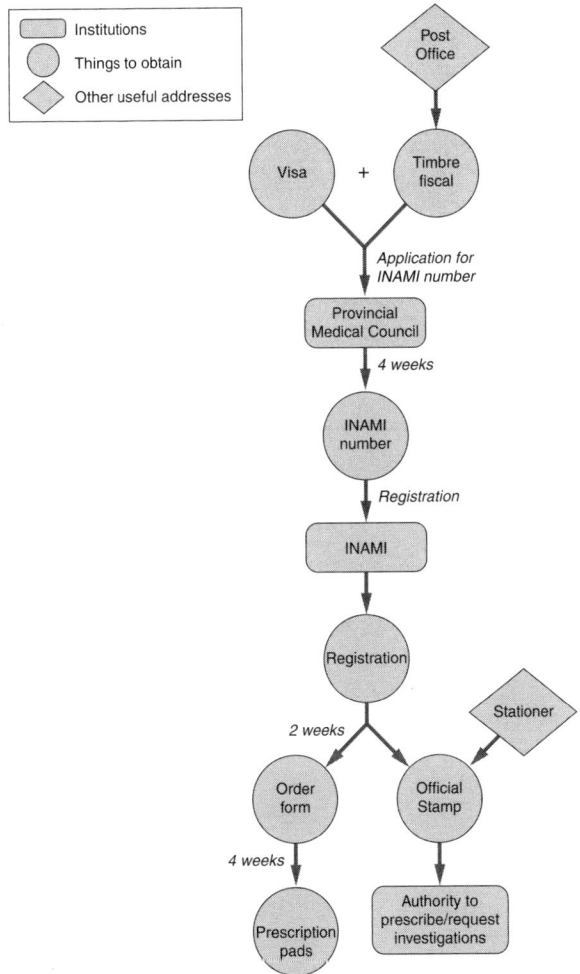

Fig. 5.2b The process of registration in Belgium.

include name, address, date of birth, qualifications, previous experience and references but little else.

After submission to the Ordre de Médecins, the documents are forwarded to the Ministry of Health for approval. The official reply must be obtained within a period of 3 months. Once this is received, one is able to contact the Commission Médicale for a visa. This can take a week or two and, once ready, it must be collected in person from the Commission Médicale. The visa is then taken, together with a post office stamp (*timbre fiscal*, available from any post office), to the Conseil Provincial de l'Ordre de Médecins for the INAMI number.

The INAMI number is issued some 4 weeks later and can be collected from the Medical Council. Before one commences practice, this number must be *registered* at INAMI. The INAMI office is on the same road, around 2 km back towards town. This final hurdle, refreshingly, takes a matter of minutes. Around a month after registration with INAMI, the doctor is issued with personalized prescription pads which can be used for outpatient prescriptions. These pads are free of charge and are delivered to the doctor's place of work.

As the INAMI number is used for everything from investigation request forms to certificates and prescriptions, it is worth ordering a stamp (*un cachet*, bought from any stationery outlet) with one's name, specialty (and/or place of work) and INAMI number. This may lessen the risk of writer's cramp from subsequent form-filling.

FINDING A POST

In Belgium, there is a high ratio of doctors to population but the distribution of doctors throughout the country is unequal, with shortages in rural and poorer areas, especially those with large immigrant populations.

It is possible for a doctor, once registered, to set up independent practice. This is not feasible for short-term stints in Belgium, though, as setting up a practice incurs considerable expense at the outset; on top of that are the costs of upkeep, and the doctor also has to establish a clientèle. Short-term placements in established practices are possible, although even GPs often work independently rather than as part of a group practice.

Posts are advertised in the medical journal of the national medical association. Often, however, posts are advertised first within each institution, as doctors who have trained as undergraduates tend to stay at the same institution for specialist training. It is useful, therefore, to contact the academic institutions directly to ascertain what posts are available and how they are to be advertised, rather than waiting for the weekly issue of the medical journal.

For jobs in francophone hospitals in and around Brussels, a monthly circular, *Ouverture de postes*, is printed by the Commission du Réseau Hospitalier Universitaire (CRHU), based at one of the main Brussels teaching hospitals. For details, contact the CRHU secretary (Tel: 02 764 5595; Fax: 02 764 5594). The CRHU is limited to hospitals affiliated to the University of Louvain, but there are several similar networks around the major universities (see List of hospitals, p. 61).

LIST OF HOSPITALS

Universitair Ziekenhuis RUG (*Flemish*)
De Pintelaan 185
9000 Gent
Tel: 00 32 (0)9 264 65 38/240 21 11

Centre Hospitalier Universitaire (*French*)
Sart Tilman
4000 Liège
Tel: 00 32 (0)4 366 7111

Clinique Universitaire de Bruxelles (*French*)
Hôpital Erasme
route Lennik 808
1070 Bruxelles
Tel: 00 32 (0)2 555 31 11
Fax: 00 32 (0)2 555 4405

Academisch Ziekenhuis (*Flemish*)
Vrije Universiteit Brussel
Laarbeeklaan 101
1090 Brussel
Tel: 00 32 (0)2 477 4111
Fax: 00 32 (0)2 477 5362

Hôpital Universitaire St Pierre (*French*)
rue Haute 322
1000 Bruxelles
Tel: 00 32 (0)2 535 3111

Hôpital Universitaire St Luc (*French*)
avenue Hippocrate 10
1200 Brussels
Tel: 00 32 (0)2 764 1111
Fax: 00 32 (0)2 764 3703

AZ Gasthuisberg (*Flemish*)
Inwendige Geneeskunde
Herestraat 46
3000 Leuven
Tel: 00 32 (0)16 34 42 59
Fax: 00 32 (0)16 34 43 07

Exchange scheme

St Luc and Gasthuisberg have been involved in the European Exchange Scheme. Contact the Professor of Medicine for further details.

ADDRESSES

Competent authority
Ordre des Médecins (*correspondence to Monsieur P.-H. Verschuren*)
Conseil National
place de Jamblinne de Meux 32
1040 Bruxelles
Tel: 00 32 (0)2 736 8291
Fax: 00 32 (0)2 735 3563

Commission Médicale du Brabant
Cité Administrative de l'État
Quartier Vesale
1010 Bruxelles
Tel: 00 32 (0)2 502 0292

Provincial Association of Doctors (*for Brussels*)
Ordre des Médecins du Brabant
avenue de Tervueren 417
1150 Bruxelles
Tel: 00 32 (0)2 771 2474

INAMI (Institut National d'Assurance Maladie-Invalidité)
avenue de Tervueren 211
1150 Bruxelles
Tel: 00 32 (0)2 739 7111
Fax: 00 32 (0)2 739 7291

British Embassy
rue Arlon 85
1040 Bruxelles
Tel: 00 32 (0)2 287 6211
Open Mon–Fri 9.30 am–12 am, 2.30 pm–4.30 pm.
A list of sworn translators is available from the British Embassy.

National formulary (*Répertoire Commenté des Médicaments*)
Centre Belge d'Information Pharmacothérapeutique
Ministère de la Santé Publique et de l'Environnement
Administration de l'Hygiène
Cité Administrative de l'État
Quartier Vesale
1010 Bruxelles
Tel: 00 32 (0)2 210 4904
Fax: 00 32 (0)2 210 4922

REGISTRABLE QUALIFICATIONS FOR BELGIAN DOCTORS GOING ABROAD

The registrable qualification awarded in Belgium is the *Diplôme légal de docteur en médecine, chirurgie et accouchements / Wetelijk diploma van doctor in de genees heel en verloskunde* (diploma of doctor of medicine, surgery and obstetrics required by law), awarded by the university faculties of medicine, the Central Examining Board or the State University Education Examining Board. The following is a list of licensing bodies (faculties of medicine) and the qualifications awarded:

- Universitaire Instelling Antwerpen: *MD Antwerp*
- Rijkuniversiteit te Gent: *MD Ghent*
- Université de l'État à Liège: *MD Liège*
- Université libre de Bruxelles ⎱ *MD Bruxelles*
- Vrije Universiteit Brussel ⎰ *MD Brussels*
- Université Catholique de Louvain ⎱ *MD Louvain*
- Katholieke Universiteit te Leuven ⎰ *MD Leuven.*

Denmark

Joined EU: 1973
Area: 43 000 km^2
Population (1998): 5.3 million
Population density: 123 persons / km^2
Language: Danish
Currency: Danish kroner
Religion: Evangelical-Lutheran (91%)
Government: Constitutional monarchy
GDP per head (1994): 19 143 US$
Social security expenditure as % of GDP (1993): 32.3%
Health expenditure as % of GDP (1995): 6.4%
Infant mortality rate (1998): 5.17 deaths per 1000 live births
Average life expectancy at birth (1998): 73.6 (men); 79.1 (women); total 76.3 years
Unemployment (1997): 7.9%
Doctors per 10 000 population (1994): 29.0
Beds per 10 000 population (1994): 5.0

BACKGROUND

Denmark is a constitutional monarchy. The single-chamber parliament (*Folketinget*) is elected on the basis of proportional representation. The present government is a social democrat-led coalition. The Danes are an extremely patriotic nation and have strong views on what they want. (Remember the unanimous rejection of the Maastricht Treaty in 1992, to the surprise of the other EU states.)

The country consists of the Jutland peninsula and numerous islands which are linked to the peninsula by road, rail and ferry. The largest of the islands is Zealand, which holds more than one-fifth of the total population. The three main cities are Copenhagen, the capital of Zealand, Århus on Jutland, and Odense where Hans Christian Andersen was born.

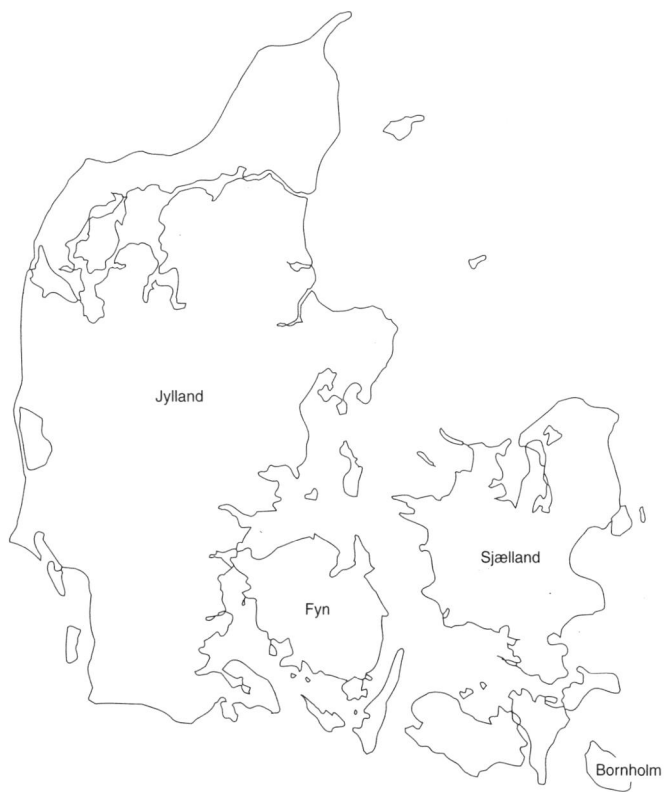

Fig. 6.1 Map of Denmark.

Greenland and the Faroe Islands are semi-autonomous members of the Danish State but do not belong to the EU. Work permits are therefore required for any individual of an EU member state who wishes to work there.

Taxation in Denmark is high but the welfare state programmes are comprehensive and efficient. Taxes are payable to both central and local government. For the latter, a tax card (*skattekort*) should be obtained from the local town hall.

Rented housing is relatively inexpensive, although often difficult to find. Most rented accommodation is unfurnished.

Cars are expensive to buy and run but there is a very good public transport system and cycling is well catered for. Since the early 1990s special tax arrangements have been made for foreigners with salaries above a certain ceiling who are working in management or in academic institutions (the *Registreringsafgift*). If these conditions apply, it is possible to buy a car without having to pay registration tax. If one ends up staying for more than 3 years, however, one must then pay back the difference.

Compulsory schooling does not start until the age of 7 years but educational standards are high.

LANGUAGE

Danish is spoken by the 5 million inhabitants of Denmark and is the official language of Greenland and the Faroe Islands, which are considered part of Denmark. Danish is one of the Scandinavian languages, a branch of the Germanic languages (part of the Indo-European family) closely related to Norwegian and Swedish.

The Danish alphabet is the same as the Norwegian, consisting of the 26 letters of the English alphabet plus æ, ø and å at the end. Before 1948, å was written aa (and is still understood in typed script, if the å character is unavailable). The spelling reforms of that year also abolished the German practice of beginning all nouns with a capital letter.

The Faroe Islands are located around 250 miles north of Scotland, midway between Norway and Iceland. Although the official language is Danish, Faroese is spoken by most of the islands' 40 000 inhabitants.

ORGANIZATION OF THE HEALTH SYSTEM

The 16 county councils, which include the city councils of Copenhagen and Frederiksberg, together with the 275 municipal councils, are responsible for management of the hospital and primary health sectors. County council responsibility is largely focused on the hospital sector and general and specialist practitioners, while primary care and much of social services administration are dealt with at municipal level. The county councils appoint health-care committees for management of regional health care. The committees are elected for a period of 4 years.

Finance

Within the Danish welfare system, the bulk of health care is financed through general taxation (85% of total health expenditure). Counties and municipalities are entitled to levy their own taxes depending on expenditure requirements. These vary according to the size of the elderly population, social requirements and so on. Of total expenditure on the health sector, around 75% goes towards the hospital sector and 25% to the primary-health sector.

Public-health schemes cover the entire population and hospital treatment is free. The standard of medical care is high. The vast majority of hospitals in Denmark are public. Private institutions account for less than 1% of total hospital beds.

During the 1980s, the total number of hospitals fell and the staff:patient ratio increased. Health-care expenditure makes up a lower share of GDP than previously but spending on primary health care has increased. Health services have recently been modelled along British NHS lines, with the emphasis on group practice and preventative medicine.

Hospital types

Hospitals can be grouped into three main categories:

- *state* and *provincial* hospitals, which have a higher percentage of specialist facilities
- *regional* hospitals, which have a certain level of specialization
- *county* hospitals, which cater for local patients.

Single-specialty hospitals exist only for psychiatry.

Hospital management

Management of hospitals is a county responsibility. Efforts are being made to offer doctors and nurses training in economics and management, to improve the relationship between political / economic and professional decision-making systems.

Access to specialist care

Denmark runs a gatekeeper system similar to that in Britain, whereby all patients must be registered with a GP and referred if specialist intervention is considered necessary. Hospital treatment is financed by the county in which a patient resides. Hospital treatment is free; charges for doctors' visits and prescriptions are refundable.

TRAINING AND TYPES OF POST

Basic medical training takes 6½ years. Following the student's graduation from medical school, the title 'doctor' can be used, but a further 18 months of pre-registration training must be undertaken. During this time the doctor can work in a subordinate position at a hospital or as a trainee in general practice. The doctor can then be registered as a physician and is permitted to practise independently as a doctor but not as a GP. Specialist training is required both for hospital specialties and for general practice. The duration of training varies, depending on specialty.

The Danish medical hierarchy is shown in Table 6.1.

Denmark	UK
Læge studerende	Student
Kursist (anyone in training)	Intern
Reservelæge	Specialist registrar
Første Reservelæge	Senior registrar
Overlæge	Consultant
Administrerende	Head of department
Cheflæge	Medical director

REGISTRATION

The competent authority is the Danish Board of Health. In order to register, one needs to obtain an application form from this board, together with a list of the documents required. Depending on EU member state of initial qualification, the standard requirements are:

- primary medical diploma
- certificate of nationality (ID certificate or passport)
- certificate of good standing (issued by the doctor's native competent authority within the last 3 months).

For nationals of Sweden or English-speaking countries, official translations of these documents are not required. Recognition of qualifications should be forthcoming within 3 months.

FINDING A POST

Vacant posts in Denmark are advertised in the weekly journal of the Danish Medical Association, *Ugeskrift For Læger* (published Friday) (see 'Addresses', below).

LIST OF HOSPITALS

Århus Kommunehospital
Nørrebrogade 44
DK-8000 Århus C
Tel: 00 45 (0)89 49 33 33
Fax: 00 45 (0)89 18 52 39

Århus Amtssygehus
 Tage Hansens Gade 2
 DK-8000 Århus C
 Tel: 00 45 (0)89 49 75 75
 Fax: 00 45 (0)89 49 72 49

Marselisborg Hospital
 P.P. Ørumsgade 11
 DK-8000 Århus C
 Tel: 00 45 (0)89 49 33 33

Skejby Sygehus
 Brendstrupgårdsvej
 DK-8200 Århus N
 Tel: 00 45 (0)89 49 55 66
 Fax: 00 45 (0)89 49 60 00

Kommunehospitalet
 Øster Farimagsgade 5
 DK-1399 København K
 Tel: 00 45 (0)33 38 33 38
 Fax: 00 45 (0)33 38 39 99

Frederiksberg Hospital
 Nordre Fasanvej 59
 DK-2000 Frederiksberg
 Tel: 00 45 (0)38 34 77 11
 Fax: 00 45 (0)38 34 77 55

Rigshospitalet (incl. Finsen)
 Administrationen, afsnit (section) 5222
 Blegdamsvej 9
 DK-2100 København Ø
 Tel: 00 45 (0)35 45 35 45
 This is Denmark's biggest hospital.

Sundby Hospital
 Italiensvej 1
 DK-2300 København S
 Tel: 00 45 (0)32 34 32 34
 Fax: 00 45 (0)32 34 39 99

Københavns Amtssygehus
 Sct. Elisabeth
 Hans Bogbinders Alle 3
 DK-2300 København S

Tel: 00 45 (0)31 55 45 00
Fax: 00 45 (0)32 84 56 54

Bispebjerg Hospital
Bispebjerg Bakke 23
DK-2400 København NV
Tel: 00 45 (0)35 31 35 31
Fax: 00 45 (0)35 31 39 99

Odense Universitetshospital
Sdr. Boulevard 29
DK-5000 Odense C
Tel: 00 45 (0)66 11 33 33
Fax: 00 45 (0)66 13 28 54

ADDRESSES

Competent authority
Danish Board of Health
Amaliegade 13
Postboks 2020
DK-1012 Copenhagen K
Tel: 00 45 (0)33 93 16 36

Danish Medical Association
Den Almindelige Danske Lægeforening
Trondhjemsgade 9
DK-2100 Copenhagen Ø
Tel: 00 45 (0)35 44 85 00; 00 45 (0)35 44 82 14 (direct)
Fax: 00 45 (0)35 44 85 05

REGISTRABLE QUALIFICATIONS FOR DANISH DOCTORS GOING ABROAD

The registrable qualification granted in Denmark is the *Bevis for bestået lægevidenskabelig embedseksamen* (diploma of doctor of medicine required by law), awarded by a university faculty of medicine, and the *Dokumentation for gennemført praktisk uddannelse* (certificate of practical training), issued by the competent authorities of the health service. There are faculties of medicine at Århus, Copenhagen and Odense (see also 'List of hospitals', above):

- Århus Universitet: *MD Århus*
- Københavns Universitet: *MD Copenhagen*
- Odense Universitet: *MD Odense*.

For further information, particularly for medical students, contact:

Royal Danish Embassy
55 Sloane Street
London SW1X 9SR
Tel: 0171 333 0200
Fax: 0171 333 0270

An information booklet, entitled 'Studying in Denmark', is available in English and Danish from the embassy.

Finland

Joined EU: 1995
Area: 337 000 km² (31 500 km² of water)
Population (1998): 5.15 million
Population density: 15 persons / km²
Languages: Finnish (93.6%); Swedish (6.3%)
Currency: Markka
Religion: Evangelical Lutheran (89%)
Government: Republic
GDP per head (1995): 15 099 US$
Health expenditure as % of GDP (1995): 7.7%
Infant mortality rate (1998): 3.82 deaths per 1000 live births
Average life expectancy at birth (1998): 73.6 (men); 80.8 (women); total 77.2 years
Unemployment (1997): 14.6%
Doctors per 10 000 population (1995): 27.7
Beds per 10 000 population (1995): 9.3

BACKGROUND

Finland is a presidential republic with a single-chamber parliament, the *Edeskunta*. The present government is a democratic-led coalition.

A large part of the country is made up of forests and lakes. The majority of the population is based in the south of the country. A Lapp population of around 2500 lives in the north.

Although part of Scandinavia, Finland used to have close economic ties with Russia, which involved trading based on timber and timber products. With the collapse of the former Soviet Union in 1991, however, Finland became obliged to join the European single market and is now probably the most Europhile of the Nordic states.

Salaries are slightly lower than those in other Nordic countries, although living expenses are high. Taxation and social security deduction are high but

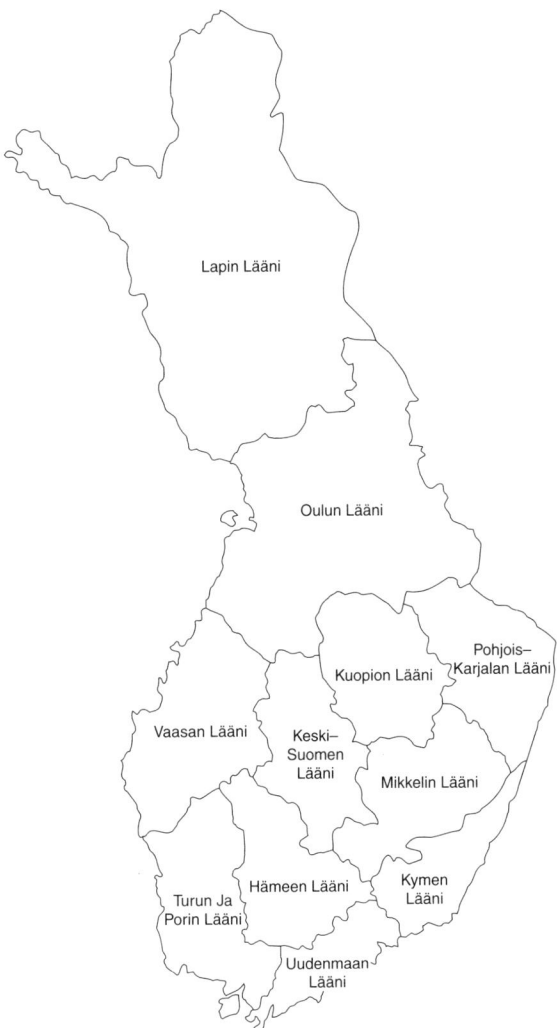

Fig. 7.1 Map of Finland.

the welfare system is well developed. On the other hand, rented property is cheaper, as is car servicing, and there is no vehicle taxation.

Residence permits are necessary for people coming to work in Finland for periods longer than 3 months. The permit is granted by the local police department. A passport or ID card is required, together with a photograph and an employment contract or other document of employment. Residence permits are granted for periods of 5 years, unless employment is of less than 1 year's duration, in which case the permit is granted only for the period of employment. Students from EEA countries are entitled to a residence permit if they are able to secure their livelihood throughout the study period.

For those driving, snow tyres are compulsory during winter months.

Education is state-provided, free and compulsory from 7–16 years.

LANGUAGE

There are around 5 million speakers of Finnish worldwide, including 70 000 in the USA. Besides being the national language of Finland, spoken by over 93% of the population, Finnish is spoken by around 200 000 people in northern Sweden and 50 000 in north-western Russia.

It is one of the Finno-Ugric languages and is difficult to learn. For example, there are 15 case forms for nouns. The alphabet consists of 21 letters: 13 consonants and 8 vowels. In principle, there is one sound for every letter and one letter for every sound. The stress is always on the first syllable.

Swedish is spoken by 6% of Finnish nationals, around 300 000 people, on the south-western and southern coasts of Finland.

Lappish is the language of the Lapps or Laplanders. These people live in northernmost Scandinavia, Finland and a small part of Russia. There are around 35 000 speakers: 20 000 in Norway, 10 000 in Sweden, 2500 in Finland and 2000 in Russia (Kola peninsula). Lappish is also one of the Finno-Ugric languages, although it is markedly different from Finnish.

ORGANIZATION OF THE HEALTH SYSTEM

As with the other Nordic countries, Finland is a welfare state. There is a comprehensive public health-care system which is supplemented by private sector providers. Social security and health-care policies are approved by the Council of State and then developed by the Ministry of Social Affairs and Health. Within this Ministry there are five main departments, dealing with administration, insurance, prevention, finance and planning, and social and health services (see Fig. 7.2). The National Board of Medicolegal Affairs (*Terveydenhuollon oikeusturvakeskus*, TEO) is part of the Department of Social and Health Affairs. TEO functions as the national competent authority and oversees the majority of health-care legislation (see Box 7.1).

State administration is represented on a local (provincial) level by the social affairs and health units of the provincial state offices in each of the 11 Finnish provinces. Within the provinces, Finland is divided into municipalities. The municipal local authorities are autonomous and deal with provision of services on a local level, according to guidelines laid down by the municipal council

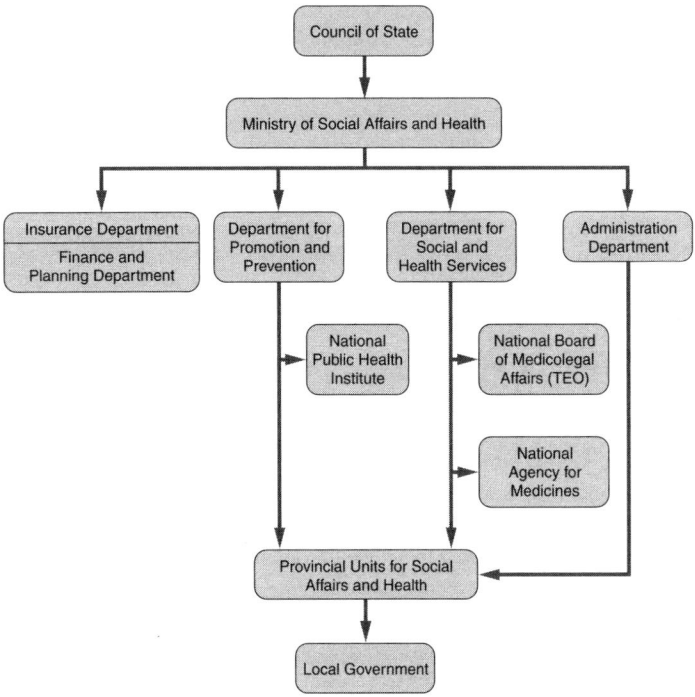

Fig. 7.2 Social welfare and health-care authorities in Finland.

BOX 7.1
The functions of TEO

Duties regarding health professionals
- Approval of education
- Recognition of primary and specialist qualifications
- Responsibility for Central Register (*TERHIKKI*)
- Discipline — in conjunction with provisional governments

Legislation regarding ethical issues
- Termination and sterilization
- Tissue transplants

Forensic duties
- Provision of places for psychiatric assessments and review of reports
- Discharge of criminal patients from mental hospitals
- Investigation into cause of death
- Assessment of injuries with respect to degree of disability

and the municipal executive board. Hospital-based services are arranged within 21 hospital districts.

Health insurance

All residents in Finland are insured against illness. Insurance premiums come from deductions from salary earners with contributions from general taxation. Permanent residents in Finland are eligible for a sickness insurance card (SII card), which can be obtained from one of the 250-odd Social Insurance Institution's local offices throughout Finland. The SII card is needed for each health-care episode at, for example, health centres, pharmacies or the SII local office.

The sickness insurance system is comprehensive but is supplemented by private sector services. Sickness insurance provides reimbursement for a proportion of the costs paid by patients to private physicians, for private examinations and for treatment and medication prescribed by a physician. Sick leave and parenthood (maternity and paternity) allowances are also provided.

All patients receiving health care or medical treatment in Finland are insured against injury resulting from such treatment, in agreement with the Patient Injury Act 1986.

Hospital types

Hospitals in Finland can be categorized according to size and degree of specialization into district and central. The municipal authorities play an important role in arranging specialist medical service provision in the former, thereby promoting a well-functioning continuum between public or primary health and specialist care in each hospital district.

There are 16 central hospitals in Finland; these are larger than the district hospitals and offer a greater range of specialties. These hospitals receive patients who are referred 'up' from district hospitals. In addition, Finland has five university hospitals which are attached to each of those universities with a faculty of medicine (see 'List of hospitals', below).

Access to specialist care

Patients requiring specialist care are referred from the municipal health clinics to specialist clinics in one of the 21 hospital districts. Referral must be to a specialist in the hospital district in which the patient is resident.

TRAINING AND TYPES OF POST

Basic medical training takes 5½ years, at the end of which the internship examination (*Pääsykoe*) is taken. After successful completion of the internship, the SHO / SpR training grade equivalent is the *apulaislääkäri*. Specialist training takes on average 6 years, although the whole process may take longer as junior doctors may have to queue for training positions. Health-care professionals are trained according to standards approved by the National Board of Medicolegal Affairs (TEO).

Once the right to specialize has been awarded, the doctor becomes an *osastonkäri* (full-time doctor) or an *erakoaskäri* (staff grade-equivalent, involved mainly in outpatient duty). The chief of service is the *ylikäri*. Licensed physicians are entitled to work independently as general practitioners after completion of a 2-year supplementary training course in basic health care.

PRACTICAL POINTS

Treatment prescription

The Ministry of Social Affairs and Health has compiled regulations on the treatment prescription of medicines, which came into effect on 1 March 1996. The Finnish reference book, *Pharmica Fennica*, is published every year. This gives details of certain pharmaceutical preparations which may only be used in hospital or prescribed by a specialist.

Legislation

TEO has a legal role in a number of ethical and forensic situations in clinical practice (see Fig. 7.2). If these situations arise, it is necessary to apply to TEO before further action can be taken. For example, TEO's permission is necessary for termination of a pregnancy after 12 weeks' gestation if for reasons other than the woman's illness or bodily injury. Even then, the limit is the 20th week of pregnancy. If the reason is fetal damage, application must always be made to TEO. In this case, permission is granted up to the end of the 24th week of pregnancy when reliable investigations have confirmed that the fetus has a severe disease or bodily defect.

Organs and tissues may be removed from a living person over 18 years of age for the treatment of another person's disease or bodily injury, for making a pharmaceutical preparation or for medical research, provided written patient consent is obtained.

For medical autopsy in the case of hospital deaths, the decision is made by the physician in charge of the unit. Consent is required by the deceased's next of kin but TEO need not be informed.

Medical defence and professional disciplinary procedures

General guidelines concerning the conduct of health-care professionals are issued by the Ministry of Social Affairs and Health. The supervision of health-care professionals is the responsibility of the provincial governments in each region in conjunction with TEO. A health professional's conduct may be inspected if a claim is made against him or her. This may result in one of three sanctions:

- *administrative control*, which is a reprimand by the authorities; the professional may be given an admonition for erroneous action
- *a disciplinary measure*, where a written caution is issued and is entered into the employee register
- *a precautionary measure*, where the right to practise a profession is limited or revoked until further notice.

The provincial government can resort only to administrative controls, whereas TEO has the authority to administer all three. TEO informs the competent authorities within the EEA of any sanctions that have resulted from the disciplinary procedure.

Private practice

TEO must be notified of self-employment by those planning to practise independently. Notification must include personal data, profession, domicile, type of self-employment and start date. TEO must also be notified of the cessation of self-employment.

For those starting a business — for example, a private health-care practice — a notification form must be sent to the National Board of Patents and Registration in order to register. The provider of services needs a permit granted by the provincial government, and appropriate facilities and personnel must be provided for, according to the Act on Private Health Care 152/90.

Insurance and pensions

Work in Finland falls under the scope of the Finnish employment pension system, except if the work assignment is short, in which case foreign citizens are usually covered by the insurance system of their country of origin. More information regarding pensions is available (in Finnish) from the Central Pension Security Institute (see 'Addresses', below).

REGISTRATION

TEO is the competent authority in Finland and recognizes primary and specialist qualifications of all medical practitioners. TEO is responsible for the

Central Register of Health-Care Professionals (*TERHIKKI*), which is maintained by the National Research and Development Centre for Welfare and Health (STAKES). Registered professionals in health care are divided into three groups: those who are licensed, those who are granted a permit, and those entitled to use a protected title. Professionals coming from EU member states may be either licensed or entitled to use a protected title. The professions for each group are listed by TEO, but as a general rule physicians or health professionals with higher degrees are licensed, whereas enrolled nurses and technicians use a protected title.

As education, including medical training, in the Nordic countries is so similar, anyone licensed in one Nordic state can be granted corresponding rights in another, according to an agreement on the joint Nordic labour market. This agreement came into effect in January 1994 and has since been revised to ensure compatibility with EU legislation.

Licensing or use of a protected title does not involve any language proficiency requirements to be confirmed by TEO. However, a certificate of language skills may be necessary, depending on the employer (the local authority).

Foreign doctors must provide evidence that their training corresponds to that received in Finland. In some cases, TEO may require professional experience, an adaption period in the profession or a qualification test before the person can be licensed or permitted to use a protected title.

To obtain registration, one needs to submit an application to TEO, specifying the profession that one wishes to practise (that is, physician, as opposed to midwife or dentist). It is recommended that the application be made in Finnish, Swedish or English. The document must be signed and dated by hand by the applicant.

Registration requires the following documents:

- passport (copy) or other certificate of nationality
- degree certificate
- valid certificate of the right to practise in one's native country (GMC certificate for UK nationals)
- certificate showing the applicant's education complies with the requirements laid down in the pertinent EU Directives. This is available from the GMC or equivalent competent authority. The document must be sent in the original and must not be more than 3 months old.

The enclosures must be officially certified copies of the original documents. Translations of the documents into Finnish, Swedish or English, made by a registered translator, must also be presented if applicable. TEO's decision on the right to practise a profession is then issued in Finnish or in Swedish and is subject to a fee of FIM400.

Once a licence to practise has been granted by TEO, one can then apply for a sickness insurance number (SV number), issued from the Social Insurance Institution (SII). The SII is informed by TEO when a licence has been granted (see 'Addresses', below).

An SV stamp can be requested at the same time from the SII. The first stamp is supplied free of charge. The SV number must be written or stamped on, for instance, all prescriptions for medications.

FINDING A POST

Posts are advertised in the journal of the Finnish Medical Association. Specialist posts are difficult to come by and Finnish nationals who have completed primary training in Finland often have to queue for positions to become available. Appointments as locum tenens are possible. It is useful to contact one of the main teaching hospitals directly (see 'List of hospitals', below).

LIST OF HOSPITALS

A complete list of hospitals in Finland is available for 100 FIM from:

Suomen kuntaliitto
2 Linja 14
FIN-00530 Helsinki
Tel: 00 358 (0)9 7711
Fax: 00 358 (0)9 771 2291

The following is a list of the five university hospitals in Finland:

Helsingen yliopistollinen keskussairaala
Stenbäckinkatu 9
FIN-00290 Helsinki
Tel: 00 358 (0)9 4711
Fax: 00 358 (0)9 471 500

Kuopion yliopistollinen sairaala
PL 1777
FIN-70211 Kuopio
Tel: 00 358 (0)17 173 311

Oulun yliopistollinen keskussairaala
PL 22
FIN-90221 Oulu
Tel: 00 358 (0)8 315 2011
Fax: 00 358 (0)8 315 4499

Tampereen yliopistollinen sairaala
Teiskontie 35
FIN-33520 Tampere
Tel: 00 358 (0)3 247 5111
Fax: 00 358 (0)3 247 5314

Turun yliopistollinen keskussairaala
Kiinamyllynkatu 4–8
FIN-20520 Turku
Tel: 00 358 (0)2 261 1611

ADDRESSES

National Board of Medicolegal Affairs (Terveydenhuollon oikeusturvakeskus, TEO)
Siltasaarenkatu 18 C, 5th floor
PO Box 265
FIN-00531 Helsinki
Tel: 00 358 (0)9 3967 280
Fax: 00 358 (0)9 3967 2842
Publishes an extremely informative 27-page document entitled 'Guide for health care professionals coming to Finland from the EU member states'. It is well worth obtaining a copy before considering a move to Finland.

Finnish Medical Association
Mäkelänkatu 2
PO Box 49
FIN-00501 Helsinki
Tel: 00 358 (0)9 393 091
Fax: 00 358 (0)9 393 0794

Social Insurance Institution
Health and Income Security Department
PO Box 78
FIN-00381 Helsinki
Tel: 00 358 (0)9 434 11
Fax: 00 358 (0)9 434 3829

Finland Trade Centre / Embassy of Finland
avenue des Arts 58
1000 Bruxelles
Tel: 00 32 (0)2 548 9600
Fax: 00 32 (0)2 548 9617
Can provide a list of the main teaching hospitals.

FINLAND

Ministry of Labour
Eteläesplanadi 4
FIN-00130 Helsinki
Tel: 00 358 (0)9 18 561
Fax: 00 358 (0)9 1856 7950
Two useful publications are available 'Are you planning to move to Finland?' (in English) and 'Tyonhakijan, ammatinharjoittajan ja opiskelijan ETA opas' (EEA guide for job-seekers, professionals and students, in Finnish).

Ministry of Social Affairs and Health
Snellmaninkatu 4–6
PO Box 267
FIN-00171 Helsinki
Tel: 00 358 (0)9 160 1
Fax: 00 358 (0)9 160 4716

National Board of Patents and Registration
Albertinkatu 25 A
FIN-00180 Helsinki
Tel: 00 358 (0)9 693 9500

Public Health Institute
Mannerheimintie 166
FIN-00300 Helsinki
Tel: 00 358 (0)9 474 41
Fax: 00 358 (0)9 474 4408

Central Pension Security Institute
Opastinsilta 7
PO Box 11
FIN-00521 Helsinki
Tel: 00 358 (0)9 1511
Fax: 00 358 (0)9 148 1172
Publishes a guide to employment pensions: 'Ulkomaalaisen työeläke Suomessa' (A foreign citizen's employment pension in Finland).

National formulary (*Therapia Fennica*)
Kandidaattikustannus Oy
Tukholmankatu 8 B
FIN-00290 Helsinki
Tel: 00 358 (0)9 241 4325

REGISTRABLE QUALIFICATIONS FOR FINNISH DOCTORS GOING ABROAD

The registrable qualification granted in Finland is the *Todistus lääketieteen lisensiaatin tutkinnosta/Bevis om medicine licential examen* (certificate of the degree of licentiate in medicine), awarded by a university faculty of medicine, *and* a certificate of practical training issued by the competent public health authorities. There are five universities with a faculty of medicine in Finland. The following is a list of these institutions and the qualifications awarded:

- Helsingin yliopisto: *Lic Med Helsinki*
- Kuopion yliopisto: *Lic Med Kuopio*
- Oulun yliopisto: *Lic Med Oulu*
- Tampereen yliopisto: *Lic Med Tampere*
- Turun yliopisto: *Lic Med Turku*.

For further information, particularly for medical students or research workers, several publications are available in English from the Finnish Institute in London at the following address:

Finnish Institute
35–36 Eagle Street
London WC1R 4AJ
Tel: 0171 404 3309
Fax: 0171 404 8893
E-mail: postmaster@finnish-institute.org.uk Website: http://www.finnish-institute.org.uk/

France

Joined EU: 1957
Area: 547 000 km^2
Population (1998): 58.8 million
Population density: 107 persons / km^2
Language: French
Currency: French franc
Religion: Roman Catholic (90%)
Government: Republic
GDP per head (1994): 17 886 US$
Social security expenditure as % of GDP (1993): 29.1%
Health expenditure as % of GDP (1995): 9.8%
Infant mortality rate (1998): 5.69 deaths per 1000 live births
Average life expectancy at birth (1998): 74.6 (men); 82.6 (women); total 78.5 years
Unemployment (1997): 12.4%
Doctors per 10 000 population (1995): 29.4
Beds per 10 000 population (1995): 8.9

BACKGROUND

France is a popular destination with British doctors because if they possess a second language that has been learnt at school, it is more likely to be French than anything else. There are nearly 2000 doctors from other EU member countries registered in France and, of these, 14 specialists and 61 generalists are from Britain. There is, however, a rising problem of unemployment and this now extends to health-care professionals.

The country is a democratic republic. This chapter deals with so-called metropolitan France, which is divided for administrative purposes into 22 *régions* (including the island of Corsica) and 96 *départements*. The Republic of France comprises metropolitan France together with ten overseas possessions, including French Guiana, Guadeloupe and Réunion.

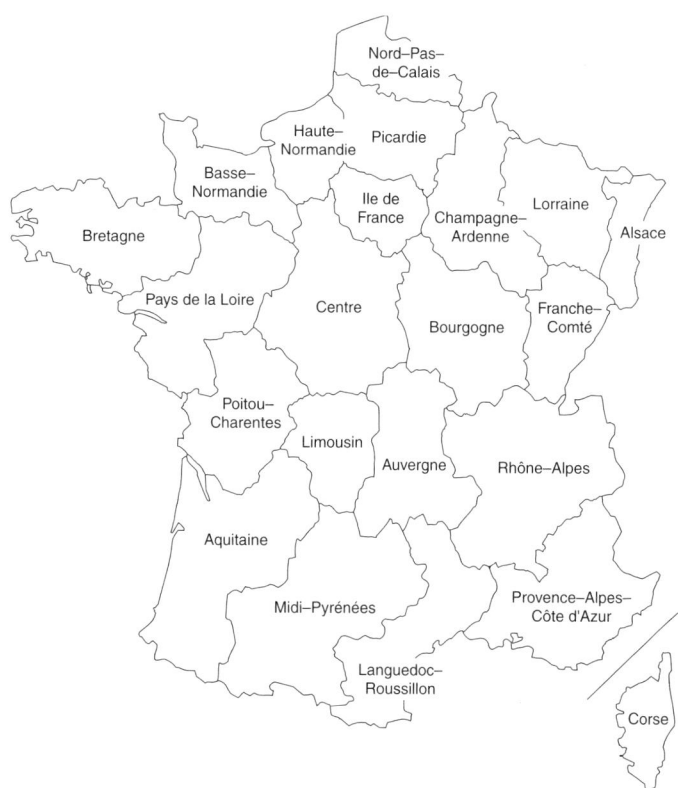

Fig. 8.1 Map of France.

Over 85% of the population are native-born. Immigrant populations are generally found in the larger cities. Around 75% of the population is urban. France and the French are quite heterogeneous, as reflected by the dialects of different regions (see 'Language', below) and the fact that registration as a medical practitioner takes place at regional rather than national level.

Employers' contributions to social security are among the highest in Europe but direct taxation is relatively low. The taxation system is very complicated. For car registration taxation, there is an additional '*circulation* tax', which varies according to *département*.

Work permits are not required for EU nationals but after 3 months of residence it is necessary to apply for a residence permit at the town hall (*la mairie*) or the police station. Such a permit may be difficult to obtain without a job.

Rents for accommodation vary depending on district. Beware the small print when renting unfurnished property.

Education is free and compulsory from 6–16 years.

LANGUAGE

There are a number of dialects spoken throughout France, although only French has official status.

Breton is spoken in Brittany, the peninsula of westernmost France between the English Channel and the Bay of Biscay. It is the only Celtic language spoken in continental Europe, the others being spoken in the UK and the Republic of Ireland. There are fewer than 1 million Breton speakers and the language is not used in schools.

Provençal, a Romance language, is spoken in Provence in south-eastern France, an area bordering Italy and facing the Mediterranean Sea.

Basque is spoken in the southwest (see Chapter 16). Catalan, another Romance language very closely related to Provençal, is spoken in a small part of France in a province of the Pyrénées-Orientales (formerly known as Roussillon). There are 250 000 speakers.

A German dialect, Alsatian, is spoken in the regions of Alsace and Lorraine (see Chapter 9).

ORGANIZATION OF THE HEALTH SYSTEM

The present social security system has been in existence since the end of the Second World War and covers health insurance, pensions, unemployment insurance and family allowances.

The French health-care system is founded on the basic principles of national solidarity and freedom of choice for both patients and doctors. Health-care provision is supported by mandatory insurance coverage and is enjoyed by over 99% of the population. Patients included in the system are entitled to see any medical practitioner of their choice as many times as they please ('medical nomadism') and a percentage of any expenses incurred is then reimbursed by their insurance funds. Doctors in turn have the freedom to practise within the state system or privately, and until recently were at liberty to investigate and prescribe at will.

This section will cover basic health-service organization at state and local level, the mechanism of patient insurance and reimbursement, the types of health care provided and the recent reforms, of which those practising in France should be aware.

The health system is highly centralized, with government control of health-care management and finance. Health policy is developed by the government and implemented by the various ministries and their regional and departmental directorates. The Ministry of Health deals with hospitals and pharmaceuticals as well as health. Policies are administered by 21 regional health offices which oversee local health-care administration. The regional offices assess local needs with a view to making recommendations to the Ministry of Health. A total of 96 provincial (local) health departments deal with primary care and serve to implement national policy regarding such issues as disease control and health education programmes. Hospital care is provided in public and private institutions. Two-thirds of the French hospital sector is public and one-third is private. Of the private hospitals, approximately half are not for profit and half are for-profit organizations. Ambulatory care is usually provided out of hospital in individually run clinics, of which 95% are private.

Finance

There are two financing mechanisms:

- Public and private *not-for-profit* hospitals receive an annual budget allocation from the State
- Private *for-profit* hospitals and *ambulatory care* organizations are paid for on a fee-for-service basis. National fee scales are set annually following negotiations between national health insurance funds (see below) and representatives of health-care professionals. The fees proposed must be approved by the Ministry of Health before being instituted.

Private practitioners are paid by insurance funds or by patients (who are then reimbursed by the insurance bodies) for services rendered. The levels of reimbursement are defined in the annual *convention médicale*.

Health insurance

Almost 95% of the population is covered by three major national health insurance funds. The largest of these, the *Caisse Nationale d'Assurance Maladie des Travailleurs Salariés*, covers around 80% of the population. This fund is restricted to salaried employees and contracts are linked to earnings and shared between employees and employers. All employed people must join either this fund or other schemes set up for particular occupations — for example, tradesmen and farmers.

The various schemes, and in particular the scheme for salaried employees, are organized on the basis of the three major administrative divisions of the country:

- At *central* level, the Caisse Nationale or National Fund coordinates activities.
- At *regional* level, the Caisse Régionale or Regional Fund controls operations.

- At *departmental* level a Caisse Primaire or Primary Fund pays out benefits.

The mandatory national funds do not cover *all* health expenditure and over three-quarters of the population subscribes to complementary private insurance schemes. There are around 6500 mutual aid funds (*mutuelles*), which are organized by professional and interprofessional branches, and around 100 private insurance companies. Resources derived from these voluntary contributions offer cover for the proportion of costs which the compulsory health insurance schemes leave to be met by the insured person.

Health insurance funds are collected by the Ministry of Social Affairs. These funds provide cover for the five major risks — old age, disability, industrial accidents, family allowances and sickness / maternity. For sickness/maternity, two types of benefit exist:

- *benefits in kind* for insured persons and their dependants in the case of medical or paramedical expenses being incurred as a result of sickness
- *cash benefits*, which provide the insured person with a replacement income in the case of absence from work.

Reforms

Health expenditure has been steadily increasing. This is owing to:

- freedom of patients regarding access to health care and of doctors regarding investigations and prescribing
- advances in medical technology, expanding the range of investigations and treatment available
- the high proportion of health expenditure which is covered by social security.

With regard to the third point, the viability of a system financed by social security contributions from working people depends on the country's economic circumstances. In periods of economic growth, health expenditure can be covered for most people. However, any downturn in economic activity, any growth in unemployment or any political incentives to reduce social security taxes will lead to diminishing financial reserves and therefore serve to amplify health-care deficits.

In 1996, health-care expenditure amounted to almost 10% of GDP. Half of the health budget was spent on hospital care and prescription costs made up almost one-fifth of spending. Many consider the French system, which allows medical nomadism of patients and which until recently had no control over treatment prescribing, to be wasteful of resources. Reforms to modify health expenditure are currently in progress.

France is pursuing two initiatives for maximizing the efficacy of health-care measures: the Conference of Consensus examines specific cases to *develop practice guidelines*, and the National Agency for the Development of Effective Medical Evaluation (ANDEM) *examines their effectiveness*. ANDEM is equivalent to the King's Fund in Britain.

The French health-care system is now undergoing its biggest shake-up since 1945 with the *Chirac–Juppé* health-care reforms. These were introduced by the previous government with the aim of limiting the increase in medical expenditure. There is a need for cultural change so that prescribers take more account of global needs when providing care for individuals. The structural reforms of the Juppé plan are founded on the hypothesis that if the quality of health care is improved, costs will fall. With these reforms, the balance of power will change, giving a stronger hand to the State in national health insurance management and making parliament responsible for setting objectives. The main features are as follows:

- There will be immediate measures to balance the health budget, such that previous health deficits will be financed over the next 12 years by a new universal tax on personal income.
- Social contributions made by working people will be extended to a universal premium.
- State control will be increased, with reorganization of national health insurance funds, so that employers gain greater representation while representation of employees will be reduced.
- Health sector accounts will be examined and expenditure limits for national insurance funds will be set.
- Hospital cost control will be decentralized, with allocation of funds for each sector by 22 new publicly owned agencies at regional level.
- Ambulatory care will be controlled by national insurance funds and government bodies.
- Gatekeeper networks will be promoted.
- Continuing medical training for health-care professionals will be made compulsory.
- Reimbursement for drugs and services will be tied to medical utility or efficacy, so that non-reimbursement will be a way to balance accounts.*

---

* Mandatory medical practice guidelines (*références médicales opposables*) were introduced in 1994 and 1995 as a means of cost containment and of standardizing patient care. For example, for ulcer treatment, it was stipulated that there would be no grounds for simultaneous prescription of two anti-ulcer drugs nor for prescribing a treatment for duodenal ulcer of greater duration than 6 weeks except when symptoms persisted. Charges for any anti-ulcer drug prescribed without such justification are not reimbursed.

These guidelines have greater implications for health-care professionals in ambulatory than in hospital care. Doctors practising outside the hospital sector who do not follow national rules for prescribing, ordering diagnostic tests and carrying out procedures will be fined.

The introduction of these guidelines as a way of limiting expenditure does have its limitations. Outcomes with respect to health-care expenditure are difficult to assess, surveillance of doctors is costly and may even outweigh the savings made, and the restrictions proposed could possibly shift expenditure from out- to inpatient services.

With regard to medical nomadism, a new system was introduced in 1997 whereby patients who consult only the GP they have selected are rewarded by being charged just one-third of the standard consultation fee. The GP later receives the balance from the health insurance branch of the social security system (popularly known as *la Sécu*). This scheme was proposed to discourage the multiple consultations with different GPs and specialists made by some patients, whilst maintaining quality of care. Doctors subscribing to this agreement cannot exceed 7500 consultations per year, as this is felt by social security not to be compatible with good-quality medical provision. The idea of encouraging gatekeeping in this way is opposed by many doctors in spite of economic logic. They argue that it is contrary to the patients' freedom to choose and perhaps they fear that their income is threatened. Certainly, independently practising specialists may suffer, as patients participating in the agreement can no longer consult spontaneously but must await GP referral.

Patient costs

Social security pays for inpatient care whatever the sector (public or private). Hospitals are paid directly by national health insurance funds at a rate of 80–100% of the total cost, depending on the age and income of the patient and the severity of the illness. There is a small *per diem* co-payment charged to the patient. If inpatient care lasts over 30 days, all subsequent charges are paid in full by social security.

Ambulatory and dental care is paid by patients at each visit. The patient is then reimbursed at around 75% of the total costs. There are co-payments for prescription drugs and medical appliances. The Ministry of Social Affairs draws up a list of drugs which are refundable and prescription co-payments run at 40–100%, according to the drug's listing and the need to prescribe it. 'Life-savers' are reimbursed at 100%.

Maternity-related care and serious or high-cost illnesses are covered completely and these patients are exempt from co-payments.

Hospital types and management

There are over 1000 public hospitals and around 2400 private hospitals in France. This amounts to around 575 000 hospital beds but because private hospitals are small, the majority of beds are within the public sector. Many of France's hospital buildings are very old but remain in operation, as they are valued as part of the country's national heritage.

Hospitals can be categorized as:

- *hospital complexes* (general and specialist)
- *rehabilitation and convalescence institutions*, which include respite beds for medium- and long-term care
- *local hospitals* or *hospital units*, which possess a minimum level of technical equipment and are situated some distance from urban centres.

Public-sector hospitals are granted legal status and financial autonomy. They are given a global state financial allocation each year as a function of their activities and this is paid to them in monthly instalments. A hospital's medical structure is organized in services. A clinical director is appointed to each, who is then responsible for the medical operation of that service. The deliberations of the hospital's board of directors are supervised by the State.

Private hospitals which are not involved in the public hospital service are not subject to the same rules and regulations. Profit-making hospitals are subject to the same regulations as commercial organizations, whether or not they have a contract with the financing bodies of the state security system. These hospitals are subject to the day rate schedule which covers operational costs, while actual medical care is paid for on a fee-for-service basis and is subject to the fee schedule drawn up by the public authorities. Private hospitals negotiate a fixed *per diem* rate annually with the government.

TRAINING AND TYPES OF POST

The education of health professionals is the responsibility of the Ministry of National Education. Medical training takes place in three stages. The first phase is open to any pupil who, on leaving school, has successfully completed the science *Baccalauréat*. There is no pre-admission interview and no other entry requirement other than the ability to cope financially. At the end of the first or second year (depending on institution), there is an examination, after which 80% of the initial intake are rejected (*numerus clausus*).

The second phase is a 4-year undergraduate training programme, involving theoretical and bedside teaching with limited ward duties. In academic teaching hospitals medical students are responsible for requesting investigations and filing results in patients' notes. They work on average from 9am to 6pm and receive a small wage.

At the end of this phase, those who pass the *Internat* examination go on to become specialists and begin the third phase of specialist training, before emerging as fully qualified specialists. Those unsuccessful in the *Internat* cannot proceed as specialists but may train in general practice. Many feel there is thus a mild stigma attached to generalists, as half of all generalists/ GPs have become so by failing the *Internat*.

Doctors are highly concentrated in urban areas and southern France compared to rural and northern regions. Almost half of all doctors are in specialist medicine and the number is rising.

Health-care professionals work in the private or public sector and either are involved in ambulatory care or are hospital-based. Hospital-based practitioners in public institutions are salaried. Ambulatory care is provided almost exclusively by private practitioners who work single-handed or in group practices and are paid on a fee-for-service basis. A small proportion of ambulatory care is provided by clinics which are run by the *départements* and employ salaried doctors on a sessional basis. For ambulatory care (general practitioners and independent specialist practitioners), practice premises are in general financed by the *Caisse Autonome de Retraite des Médecins Français* (CARMF) and trade union institutions, or through private sources.

Hospital doctors' titles are as follows:

- *Attaché (e)* — part-time
- *Remplaçant(e)* — locum
- *Assistant(e)* — posts of 1–6 years maximum (part of training programme)
- *Practicien hospitalier* — permanent post, for which it is necessary to sit an examination (*le concours*) appropriate to the chosen discipline, organized each year by the Health Minister.

In General practice, all doctors are included in the nationally agreed fees *Convention* of 1990 unless they exercise their right to withdraw. There are three options:

- Practitioners may choose not to participate in the *Convention*. In this case, fees are unlimited but patients who consult these doctors receive only a small partial reimbursement of fees charged, although prescriptions are reimbursed normally. Only 3% of all doctors have withdrawn from the *Convention*.
- Practitioners may choose to be covered by sector 1 of the *Convention*. This obliges them to charge the fees agreed in the tariff negotiations and patients are then reimbursed.

- Practitioners may choose sector 2 of the *Convention*, and be permitted to charge moderately higher fees.

All doctors who accept the *Convention* are private doctors. Private practitioners are subject to all the regulations of the *Code de la Santé Publique*, the Code of Ethics and all regulations governing medical practice in France.

PRACTICAL POINTS

Insurance and pensions

All doctors in practice have to join the superannuation scheme, CARMF, which provides a pension from age 65 if the doctor decides to retire, and insurance in case of illness, invalidity or death. Sickness insurance within the social security system is obligatory. It can be augmented by private insurance, as described above (see 'Health insurance').

Medical defence and professional disciplinary procedures

Although doctors are not required to be insured for professional liability, most of them do so. In France, arrangements for professional cover are made mainly by the insurance company *Le Sou Médical*. This company provides legal advice and services where appropriate. The national competent authority (*Ordre des Médecins*) is responsible for professional discipline, and in the event of serious charges the doctor may appear in the civil or criminal courts of law. Settlements for malpractice complaints are often reached between patients and insurance companies rather than bringing the doctor(s) involved to court individually.

Post-mortem examinations

According to legislation passed in 1976, post-mortem examination was able to be performed except if the patient or family specifically expressed opposition before the patient's death. New legislation in 1994 made distinctions between the removal of organs for therapeutic transplants, post-mortem examination for scientific research and teaching, and that for determining the cause of death.

REGISTRATION

The competent authority is the *Conseil National de l'Ordre des Médecins*. Registration applications should be addressed to the President of the Council of the departmental Council or *Ordre* in which the doctor wishes to practise.

When a doctor is inscribed on the *Tableau de l'Ordre* by the departmental Council, he or she is listed either with doctors qualified in general medicine (generalists) or with specialist doctors of the relevant specialty. A doctor may mention only one specialty on his or her professional logo on prescription forms and in a directory.

For GPs, the practice is submitted for inscription on the list of the Ordre des Médecins, provided the GP is an EU citizen and has trained in an EU member state.

Registration is relatively simple for nationals of the European Economic Area. It is best to apply initially to the national Ordre des Médecins, however, as the requirements differ for each country. Some examples are given in Box 8.1.

BOX 8.1
Registration procedures in France

- For doctors native to Germany, Spain, Greece, Italy, Luxembourg and Portugal, the application must be accompanied by a certificate from the member state that has delivered the diploma confirming that every condition foreseen by EU obligations has been met.
- If training has been completed before 1 January 1991 for Greece or before 1 January 1986 for Spain, the application must be accompanied by a certificate from the competent authority of the member state stating that the doctor has been practising for at least 3 consecutive years within the 5 years preceding the date of the certificate.
- For doctors native to former East Germany, a similar certificate is required for training completed before 3 October 1990, and training before this time has to be approved.
- For EFTA countries and for countries joining the EU after 1995, the primary qualification diploma must be accompanied by a certificate of practical training awarded by the national competent authority. Note that, for Austria, the certificate mentioned (*Bescheinigung über die Absolvierung der Tätigkeit Arzt im Praktikum*) has never existed and so the basic diploma is thus sufficient.

In general, the following documents are required:

- certified copy of the basic medical diploma (qualification); a list of the relevant diplomas for each country is provided by the Ordre des Médecins and is the same as that listed at the end of each country chapter in this book
- birth certificate or a statement of civil status issued not more than 3 months previously
- certificate of nationality (passport or identity card)

- extract from police records (*Extrait du casier judiciaire*) or equivalent document giving details of any criminal offence, or a certificate of good standing from the competent authority, which must have been issued within 3 months of the application
- sworn statement by the applicant that there are no proceedings pending against him or her or matters which could give rise to any disciplinary condemnation or sanction or affect his or her registration
- evidence of some form to establish that the applicant has a sufficient knowledge of the French language.

The relevant documents must be translated by a recognized translator (*traducteur agréé*). Addresses of these are available from the British Embassy in Paris or from the Berlitz School of Translators in London (see p. 211 for address). Once a completed application file has been received, the departmental Council will make a decision within a maximum period of 3 months. This is for recognition both of the primary qualification of medicine and of registration as a medical practitioner in the doctor's native country. Once *recognition* is obtained, obtaining full *registration* and inscription on the list of the regional competent authority takes a little longer.

Before starting practice, the doctor also has to register the diploma of medicine at the headquarters (*préfecture*), at the *Direction Départementale de l'Action Sanitaire et Sociale* (DDASS), and with the Clerk of the Court of First Instance (addresses from the regional competent authority). Such registration must be carried out within 1 month of establishment.

DELF and DALF

The *Diplôme d'Études en Langue Française* (DELF) and the *Diplôme Approfondi de Langue Française* (DALF) are official examinations in French as a foreign language. They are recognized by the French Ministry for Education for academic and professional purposes. They are similar to the IELTS examination in the UK (see p. 211) in that they are not required for citizens of EU member states for recognition of primary qualifications but may be necessary for entry in to certain university courses. It is necessary to have the DELF first before being eligible to sit the DALF, which examines proficiency in French to a higher level.

The Anglo-French Medical Society (AFMS)

AFMS was inaugurated in 1983. It is closely affiliated with the *Association Médicale Franco-Britanique* and aims to promote the mutual exchange of medical experience and knowledge, cooperation and education. Scientific meetings have been held since 1984 between British and French doctors on both sides of the Channel.

For medical students, the Society provides a number of scholarships each year for medical electives to francophone institutions.

Since 1994, an excellent French language course has been running from the University of Liverpool. The course is held on weekends in January. Details are available from the Department of Medicine at the Royal Liverpool University Hospital. The British Medical Association International Department can provide the address of the Society's president for further information. (This is not provided here as it is subject to change.)

FINDING A POST

The following may be useful:

- Consulting the medical press: *Le Concours médical*, *La Revue du praticien* and *Le Médecin de France* are the leading medical journals.
- Contacting the medical institution in which one would like to work. Contact can be either with medical personnel (*bureau du personnel médical*) or with the head of the relevant department. This is recommended, as not all vacant posts are advertised in journals.
- *Directions régionales des affaires sanitaires et sociales* (DRASS), which provides a list of vacant posts in public institutions and a list of hospital establishments in general. (The address is available from the competent authority once registration has been obtained).

There is open competition for vacancies that are advertised. Information on vacancies for salaried doctors is available from DDASS which is based in the departmental *préfecture*.

Doctors wishing to set up *independent* practice have no restrictions placed on them other than the law of supply and demand. The medical press gives indications of appropriate areas for setting up in practice.

There are literally thousands of hospitals in France, distributed throughout the various regions and departments. While considering a job, therefore, it is advisable first to consider the region in which one would like to work. The next step is then to contact some of the hospitals in this area to ask when jobs are likely to be available and how to apply. As medical registration is regional, it is better to have an idea of where the future post is likely to be located before beginning the registration procedure.

LIST OF HOSPITALS

I have not listed many hospitals in France, as a full list would require a second volume of this book. A comprehensive list is, however, available in the

Guide Rosenwald (Annuaire du corps médical français; 1997, 110th edition), a large, red book in two volumes. Volume I deals with administration and social security and gives addresses of universities, laboratories and professional organizations. Volume II is more useful: part 1 provides details of all registered hospitals in France, according to area (*Classement géographique des établissements hospitaliers publics et privés*); parts 2–4 deal with all registered doctors, according to region. The list is divided into those who are hospital-based and, of non-hospital doctors, those who are generalists or specialists. This book is available in the French Embassy of most countries and in large libraries. It is the definitive reference but the reader should beware of advertisements; given that a fair number of hospitals are private, a large entry in the hospital directory does not necessarily indicate a well-reputed academic institution. It can equally be a large private concern that can afford to pay for advertising space with its profits.

Hôpital de l'Institut Pasteur
209–211 rue de Vaugirard
75015 Paris
Tel: 00 33 (0)1 40 61 38 00
Fax: 00 33 (0)1 40 61 38 79
Number of beds: 60.

American Hospital of Paris
63 boulevard Victor Hugo
(Entrée 84 boulevard de la Saussange)
92202 Neuilly sur Seine
Tel: 00 33 (0)1 46 41 25 25; 00 33 (0)1 46 41 27 27 (Welcome service)
Fax: 00 33 (0)1 46 24 49 38
Number of beds: 110 surgical, 44 medical, 18 obstetric, 7 cardiac / high dependency, 8 intensive care.

European Exchange Scheme

Groupe hospitalier Necker — Infants Malades
Départment de Nephrologie
149 rue de Sèvres
75743 Paris Cedex 15
Tel: 00 33 (0)1 44 49 40 00 } General
Fax: 00 33 (0)1 44 49 40 90
Tel: 00 33 (0)1 44 49 54 11 } Renal unit
Fax: 00 33 (0)1 44 49 54 50

ADDRESSES

Competent authority
Conseil National de l'Ordre des Médecins
180 boulevard Haussmann
75389 Paris Cedex 08
Tel: 00 33 (0)1 53 89 32 00
Fax: 00 33 (0)1 53 89 32 01

Ambassade de France
42 boulevard du Régent
1000 Bruxelles
Tel: 00 32 (0)2 548 8711
Open 9.30 am–11.30 am, 2.30 pm–4 pm. The French Embassy in Brussels holds a copy of the Guide Rosenwald *and the staff are helpful.*

Assistance Publique des Hôpitaux de Paris (*deals with numerous establishments*)
3 avenue Victoria
75004 Paris
Tel: 00 33 (0)1 40 30 27 00

Confédération des Syndicats Médicaux Français (*closest equivalent to BMA*)
60 boulevard de Latour-Maubourg
75340 Paris Cedex 07
Tel: 00 33 (0)1 47 05 59 72
Fax: 00 33 (0)1 45 51 82 13

Médecins sans Frontières (UK)
124–132 Clerkenwell Road
London EC1R 5DL
Tel: 0800 731 6746

REGISTRABLE QUALIFICATIONS FOR FRENCH DOCTORS GOING ABROAD

The registrable qualifications granted in France are the *Diplôme d'État de docteur en médecine* (State diploma of doctor of medicine), awarded by the university faculties of medicine, the university joint faculties of medicine and pharmacy, or by the universities; and the *Diplôme d'université de docteur en médecine* (University diploma of doctor of medicine), where that diploma certifies completion of the same training course as that laid down for the state diploma of doctor of medicine.

There are 33 universities with faculties of medicine, of which 6 are in Paris. The following list gives examples of licensing bodies (faculties of medicine) and the qualifications awarded:

- Université de Grenoble: *MD Grenoble*
- Université de Lille II: *MD Lille*
- Université de Paris (V, VI, VII, XI, XII and XIII): *MD Paris*.

Further information on France, particularly for medical students, is available from the following sources:

French Institute
17 Queensberry Place
London SW7 2DT
Tel: 0171 838 2148
Fax: 0171 838 2145

French Embassy Cultural Department
23 Cromwell Road
London SW7 2El
Tel: 0171 838 2055
Fax: 0171 838 2088

Germany

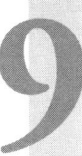

Joined EU: 1957
Area: 357 000 km²
Population: (1998): 82.1 million
Population density: 230 persons / km²
Language: German
Currency: Deutschmark
Religion: Protestant (majority Lutherans, 38%); Roman Catholic (34%); Muslim (2.5%)
Government: Federal republic
GDP per head (1994): 18 326 US$
Social security expenditure as % of GDP (1993): 29.7%
Health expenditure as % of GDP (1995): 10.4%
Infant mortality rate (1998): 5.2 deaths per 1000 live births
Average life expectancy at birth (1998): 73.8 (men); 80.3 (women); total 77 years
Unemployment (1997): 12%
Doctors per 10 000 population (1994): 33.6
Beds per 10 000 population (1994): 9.7

BACKGROUND

The 1990s have seen fundamental changes in the structure of Germany since the reunification of east and west in October 1990. Germany is now the largest EU country and has the highest number of doctors, dentists, pharmacists, hospital beds and medical equipment.

The country is a federal republic of 16 states (*Länder*). There are 13 federal states and 3 city states of Berlin, Hamburg and Bremen. There is a President and a two-house parliament. The seat of government is currently in Bonn, the capital of the old Federal Republic (West Germany), but was due to move to Berlin in the year 2000.

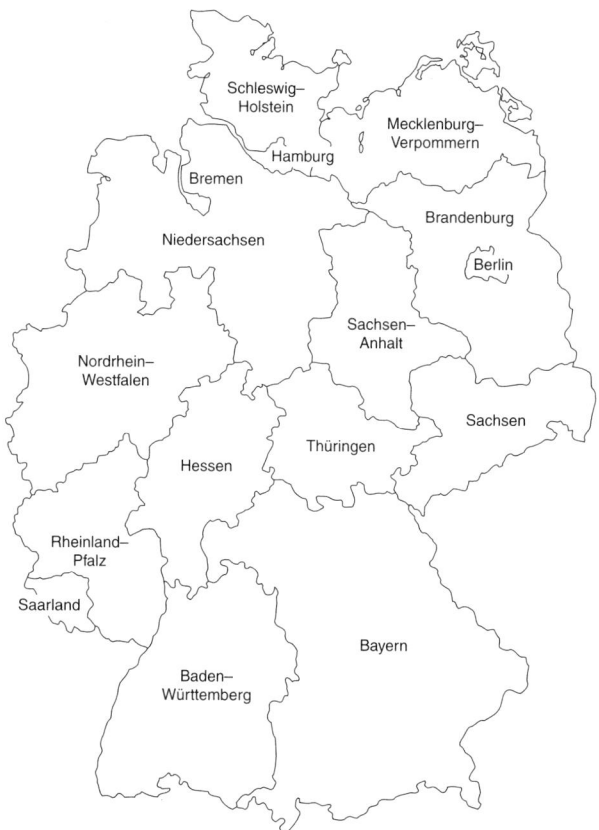

Fig. 9.1 Map of Germany.

There are 7.2 million non-German residents in Germany, of which 116 000 are British. The population density in the western regions is high, exceeded by only Belgium, the Netherlands and Britain. Former East Germany is less densely inhabited, with less than one-fifth of the total population. The number of doctors per head of population is the fourth highest in the EU. Unemployment is high, with 11 000 doctors registered unemployed, predominantly in the hospital sector.

Income tax is levied on a graduated scale and a percentage of employees' salaries goes towards sickness insurance, pensions and unemployment benefit. A solidarity tax of 5.5% is a recent development. Married couples can file a joint tax return, even if only one partner has an income. Tax is higher than in Britain, but lower if married or with children. There is no car registration tax.

A residence permit (*Aufenthaltserlaubnis*) is required for stays longer than

3 months for EEA nationals, available from the Foreign Nationals authority at the local town hall or area administrative centre. These are renewable every 5 years.

Education is compulsory from 6–18 years.

LANGUAGE

German is a Germanic language like English and Dutch. It is widely spoken throughout Europe. As well as being the national language of Germany and Austria and one of the four official languages of Switzerland, German is spoken in the Alsace-Lorraine region of France, in the Alto-Adige region of Italy, in Luxembourg, Liechtenstein and the eastern cantons of Belgium.

Between these regions the spoken dialects vary considerably, although the written language is quite uniform. Two dialect divisions are often referred to. High German or *Hochdeutsch* is spoken in the highlands of the south and is the standard written language. Low German or *Plattdeutsch*, spoken in the lowlands of the north, is more commonly spoken and sounds more akin to English or Dutch.

The German alphabet contains the additional letter β (double s), used in the lower case.

ORGANIZATION OF THE HEALTH SYSTEM

Health insurance

Germany was the first country to develop a national insurance system for health care. The scheme was introduced by Bismarck in 1883 with the passing of the Sickness Insurance Act. Following the Act, sickness funds which had been present for high wage-earners had to take on cover for low wage-earners and the sick.

There are now around 1200 sickness funds. Insurance payments are based on a percentage of income, split between employers and employees. The system is based on solidarity, so that high income-earners contribute to low wage-earners and the well pay for the sick.

Health insurance can broadly be classified into statutory and private. Blue-collar workers below a certain income bracket are required to join one of the statutory sickness funds. There are particular insurance funds for certain occupations so that, for example, agricultural workers must join one of the *Landwirtschaftliche Krankenkassen* and sailors must join the *Seekrankenkasse*.

The majority of the population is insured with the *GKV* (*Gesetzliche Krankenversicherung*), which is a type of statutory health insurance. The statutory insurance scheme covers groups such as the unemployed, students and the disabled, and the insured individual's family members also receive benefits.

Employees with higher incomes may join the *GKV* voluntarily or opt out. Private schemes operate in parallel, providing full cover for those who opt out of the statutory scheme, or complementary cover for those within it. Salaried employers and the self-employed earning more than a statutory ceiling can enrol with one of the private insurance companies, of which there are around 40. Private insurance provides more freedom of choice for those covered but there are certain drawbacks. Such insurance is expensive and premiums are higher for those with families or previous ill health. Once one has taken out private insurance, it is not possible to switch back to the statutory sickness scheme unless one's salary has fallen into the appropriate income bracket.

East Germany

The health system of the former East Germany differed from that of the West in terms of funding and emphasis on primary care. Health care was publicly funded by taxation revenue. There was a strong emphasis on prevention, with ambulatory health centres (polyclinics) and occupational services. Problems with this system included lack of resources, inflexibility and the fact that planning did not meet changing demands and budgets were not distributed according to usage patterns.

The polyclinics were given 5 years' grace after unification but were quickly disbanded as physicians began to set up private practice. Sickness funds began to operate throughout Germany in January 1991 and health-care organization is now more or less uniform.

Finance

Medical services can be divided into ambulatory and inpatient care. The former is a private set-up, with physicians working in individual practices rather than groups and earning on a fee-for-service basis. Around 60% of ambulatory care doctors are specialists, with the remainder being GPs. Patients are free to consult any specialist of their choice as an outpatient and fees are met by the sick funds. Doctors who care for sickness fund-insured patients must by law belong to a regional physician association, of which there are over 20 nationwide. Fees are negotiated between the sick fund associations and the representative body of physicians and are set within each federal state. Fees charged to privately insured patients are permitted to be higher but even these fees cannot exceed an agreed percentage of the statutory charge. As the fee per patient visit is low, ambulatory care physicians augment their incomes by organizing a battery of investigations for their patients and prescribing treatments. This is a source of waste within the health service, as patients who are then admitted to hospital are often reinvestigated.

Hospital treatment is paid directly by the insurance funds, with patients paying a nominal daily fee. University hospitals (see below) receive contributions for teaching medical students and training junior doctors. As hospitals are paid per patient day rather than by services provided, and as investigations are generally performed in the initial acute period, long-stay patients are economically attractive as they cost the same as brief acute admissions. There is thus little incentive for early discharge. The idea of convalescence is something not seen in all EU countries. Patients who have recently been hospitalized are entitled to periods of convalescence — for example, in spa centres. The entitlement for health spa attendance used to be for a maximum of 4 weeks once every 3 years. Since the health reforms of 1995, however, many services previously available on health insurance have been withdrawn and costs are now shared by the patient.

Hospital types

Since reunification, hospitals have decreased in number because of hospital planning in the new *Länder*. Nevertheless, there are still around 3500 hospitals in Germany, not counting rehabilitation centres, most of which are general. Just under half of these are state-run, providing over 60% of general hospital beds. Religious and other not-for-profit organizations like the German Red Cross run charitable hospitals, which provide around one-third of hospital beds. There are numerous private hospitals in the former West Germany but these tend to be low-capacity and so make up a relatively small contribution to total hospital beds.

Hospitals can be categorized as follows:

- *Univeristätskliniken* — university hospitals
- *Lehrkrankenhäuser* — teaching hospitals
- *Kreiskrankenhäuser* — district hospitals
- *Rehabilitationskliniken* — rehabilitation hospitals.

Access to specialist care

Patients may register with any doctor of their choice. There is no gatekeeper system, so that access to specialist care as an outpatient does not require referral. Patients insured under the statutory insurance scheme now pay a fixed contribution towards prescription costs and a fixed co-payment for periods spent in hospital. Exemptions exist for those aged under 18 years, the unemployed and other low-income populations. Refunds for charges made for non-German residents are possible by exchanging a Form E111 for a *Krankenschein* certificate issued by the German health insurance companies through the local Sickness Fund.

Patients are free to select any hospital for this specialist advice but admission requires referral. Waiting lists are few, but if patients present directly to a hospital they can be admitted without referral. Nearly half of all admissions occur in this way; around one-fifth of these are emergencies.

As German citizens are entitled to consult any specialist of their choice at any time, there is little interest in primary care. Before unification, primary care in erstwhile East Germany was provided in community-based polyclinics but these have been phased out since 1995 and replaced by independent practices. There are presently no plans for a gatekeeper system.

TRAINING AND TYPES OF POST

Undergraduate training at university is for a minimum of 6 years. Basic science is studied for the first 3 and then clinical studies for the second 3. Only the final year involves daily ward work. In this final year (the *Praktisches Jahr*), students have 4-month attachments in a medical and a surgical specialty and then 4 months in a specialty of their choice.

At the end of the 6 years, the students must pass the *Staatsexamen*. As part of this passing-out examination, most students also submit a project and have to sit a viva (oral examination). Following graduation, the successful candidate is entitled to practise medicine but cannot use the title of *Doktor* unless he or she has an MD/PhD equivalent. The title used instead is *Arzt*. In order to use the title of Doctor of Medicine (*Doktortitel*), if eligible, one has to apply to the competent *Landesminister*.

The PRHO equivalent is the *Arzt im Praktikum*. Doctors in training must work for 18 months if they wish to practise medicine. The salary at this level is considerably lower than for the equivalent in Britain (compare with *Assistanzarzt* level, p. 107). At the end of this period, the *Approbation* is awarded (the equivalent of full registration). The *Approbation* can be undertaken in the chosen specialty (in medicine, surgery, anaesthetics and so on).

Training after obtaining the *Approbation* in general internal medicine takes 6 years, in approved posts (and can include the time spent as an *Arzt im Praktikum*). Approved posts may be in almost any type of hospital but at least 1 year must be spent with a recognized teaching physician and at least 4 years on the wards, ideally including 6 months in intensive care. (See below for the body in charge of recognizing approved posts.) The title *Facharzt für Innere Medizin* is then awarded after an oral examination, the *Fachgespräch*, is passed. This is the equivalent to obtaining a Certicate of Completion of Specialist Training (CCST) in general medicine.

Training in a medical specialty must include at least 2 years of general training, of which 1 year must be completed after the *Facharzt für Innere Medizin* has been awarded. The minimum total training period for a specialty is 5 years. During this time, the trainee must keep a logbook of practical procedures and investigations performed. Note that certain medical subspecialties — for example, neurology and dermatology — are not included in general internal medicine and so general medical training in this case is not required.

The curriculum for specialist training is set by the regional chamber of physicians (*Landesärztekammer*). This body is also responsible for the final examination of undergraduates and for the awarding of specialist status. Although there are some regional variations, the curriculum is broadly similar throughout the country.

Hospital doctors' titles are as follows:

- *Stationsarzt* — ward physician
- *Assistanzarzt* — specialist registrar
- *Oberarzt* — senior registrar/junior consultant
- *Chefarzt* — head of department.

Only the specialist qualification in general internal medicine is directly transferable. For British trained doctors, only training completed after the MRCP (UK) can be counted towards training in a medical sub-specialty, and *prior* approval should be obtained from the appropriate Royal College.

From the year 2005, GP training will be of 5 years' duration postregistration rather than the current 3 years. This is according to a bill passed in June 1997, which aimed to boost flagging public confidence in GPs.

PRACTICAL POINTS

Terms and conditions

Contracts usually include a probationary period in which either party can terminate the contract at 2 weeks' notice. After this, contracts are given for 1–3 years. Study leave is less plentiful but is variable, depending on the type of institution.

Conditions of employment are available from the Marburger Bund, the German junior doctors' trade union. The average basic salary at *Assistanzarzt* level is higher than in Britain, and there are married persons' and child supplements. Additional duty hours and on-call work are paid, depending on how onerous the particular on-call duty is.

Insurance and pensions

Superannuation contributions are compulsory and made to a state-run pension fund for doctors (*Ärztliche Versorgungswerke*). The address of the regional pension scheme is available from the Bundesärztekammer. Funds cannot be transferred to the UK on return, but could be reserved until retirement age in Germany.

Medical defence and professional disciplinary procedures

Medical indemnity cover is often provided by the hospital; however, insurance companies exist for professional liability (e.g. Medical Protection Society, address below). Who provides cover should be ascertained before taking up practice.

Private practice

German doctors working in the social security system are allowed to consult privately, and it is possible to do so exclusively. Practice premises have to be maintained and financed by the individual doctor, however, and raising the necessary capital can be difficult. Professional cooperative societies exist which provide credits but are also available to give advice. The regional associations of sickness fund physicians are not permitted to refuse admission to a qualified physician, as this is seen as inhibiting the doctor's right to earn a living. However, admission can be denied if there is an excess of over 50% of doctors in a specific specialty. There are indirect ways to discourage admission to over-subscribed areas, including denial of bank loans in areas with surplus doctors and provision of low-interest loans in areas with shortages.

REGISTRATION

There are rather a lot of places to contact and information to gather when tackling registration in Germany. To make matters slightly clearer, the following is a suggestion of how to get through the necessary practicalities.

First find a post, either through advertisements or by writing directly to the head of department in a suitable hospital. Next, contact the German medical association, the *Bundesärztekammer* (see 'Addresses' below). This body can supply you with all the information you need in order to become registered and can help with finding posts or supplying a list of the main hospitals. You can obtain details of registration for certain temporary posts (i.e. whether or not registration would be required) and a list of the addresses of all necessary bodies in the various *Länder* (see Box 9.1)

Having armed yourself with a list of the authorities to contact, tackle the next steps:

- Obtain *Approbation* from the regional authority. Application is made to the regional authority of the *Land* in which the post is based. (See Box 9.2

> **BOX 9.1**
> **Useful addresses available from the Bundesärztekammer**
>
> - Regional authorities — for recognition of primary medical qualification, necessary for *Approbation*
> - Regional associations of panel doctors — for permission to practise in the social security system
> - Regional Ärztliche Versogungswerke — obligatory pension scheme for medical doctors
> - Regional Ärztekammern — membership obligatory in order to practise; the regional Ärztekammer is also responsible for recognition of post-graduate specialist training

> **BOX 9.2**
> **Application for Approbation**
>
> The following documents are likely to be required:
>
> - medical diploma of primary qualification
> - birth certificate (and marriage certificate, where applicable)
> - passport or other proof of nationality
> - curriculum vitae with photograph
> - certificate from competent authority (GMC for British doctors)
> - certificate of good standing (issued by competent authority and valid for 3 months)
> - certificate of good conduct, issued by the police
> - personal declaration that there are no legal proceedings against the applicant
> - medical certificate confirming sufficient physical and mental state to practise
>
> These items should be translated into German by a registered translator and sent, together with the original documents, to the regional chamber of physicians (Landesärztekammer) of the *Land* in which employment is to be based.

for a list of the documents required.) If rendering only temporary service, EEA nationals do not need an *Approbation*. It is advisable to write to the Bundesärztekammer, however, to ensure approval of temporary status.

- Register with the regional panel of physicians (*Ärztekammer*). Once the *Approbation* has been obtained, registration is dealt with by the Ärztekammer of the relevant *Land*. To register, there is a basic initial fee and then annual fees. The latter vary from *Land* to *Land* and in some cases according to income.
- If wishing to practise independently, register with the regional *Kassenärztliche Vereinigung* and then obtain permission to practise in the

social security system from the regional *Zulassungsausschuss* (registration committee). For independent medical practice accepting social security patients, the doctor must inform the regional Kassenärztliche Vereinigung of the relevant *Land* (see Box 9.3 for requirements). The membership fee is a small percentage of the gross income. On receipt of the *Approbation*, permission is required to practise in the social security system, and this is obtainable from the regional Zulassungsausschuss (see Box 9.4).

BOX 9.3
Registration with the Kassenärztliche Vereinigung (for independent practice)

This requires the following documents:

- *Approbation*
- birth certificate (and marriage certificate, if applicable)
- certificate of higher academic qualification (MD / PhD), if appropriate
- GP or specialist accreditation (must be recognized by the regional Ärztekammer)
- evidence of medical posts held since qualification

BOX 9.4
Permission to practise in the social security system (for independent practice)

The following must be presented:

- copy of Kassenärztliche Vereinigung registration (recognized nationally)
- evidence of medical posts held post-qualification
- curriculum vitae
- certificate of good conduct (see Box 9.2)
- details of current employment
- declaration stating you have not been drug- or alcohol-dependent in the past 5 years
- certificate of attendance at an introductory course arranged by the Kassenärztliche Vereinigung within the preceding 4 years

---

Proof of language competence is not required and it is up to the employer to ensure that the applicant has the appropriate language skills.

FINDING A POST

Salaried positions, including hospital posts, are advertised in the regional journals of the Ärztekammer or in the *Deutsches Ärzteblatt*, a weekly journal published by Deutscher Ärzteverlag (address below). Details of posts are also held by the *Zentralstelle für Arbeitsvermittlung* (address below).

Vacant posts are often filled without advertising and so a better strategy is often to write directly to the head of department (*Chefarzt*) in whatever specialty you would like to work, enclosing a CV and copies of qualifications, preferably translated into German. (These documents can then be reused for registration if you get the job.)

LIST OF HOSPITALS

A list of university hospitals is available from:

Deutsche Krankenhausgesellschaft
Tersteegenstrasse 9
D-40474 Düsseldorf
Tel: 00 49 (0)211 454 73 0
Fax: 00 49 (0)211 454 73 61

Exchange scheme

Medizinische Hochschule Hannover
Abteilung Nephrologie
Carl-Neuberg-Strasse 1
D-30625 Hannover
Tel: 00 49 (0)511 532 23 94
Fax: 0049 (0)511 55 23 66

ADDRESSES

Bundesärztekammer (*German medical association*)
Herbert-Lewin-Strasse 1
D-50931 Köln
Tel: 00 49 (0)221 40 04 0
Fax: 00 49 (0)221 40 04 388 / 384
Supraregional body; supplies list of regional authorities for Approbation application, regional Ärtzekammer for registration, regional Kassenärztliche Vereinigung for establishment as a free-practising doctor; also provides curriculum for specialist training, approves specialist posts, and is in charge of final examinations and awarding specialist status. (The latter must then be recognized by the regional Ärztekammer.)

Marburger Bund (*German junior doctors' trade union*)
Riehler Strasse 6
D-50668 Köln
Tel: 00 49 (0)221 973 1670

Zentralstelle für Arbeits vermittlung
Feuerbachstrasse 42
D-60325 Frankfurt
Website: www.arbeitsamt.de

Deutsches Ärtzeblatt
Published weekly by Deutscher Ärtzteverlag
Dieselstrasse 2
D-50859 Köln
Tel: 00 49 (0) 2234 7011 120
Fax: 00 49 (0)2234 7011 142
Website: www.aerzteblatt.de.
Details of this journal are also available from the Bundesärtzekammer or it can be accessed on the Internet (http://www.aerzteblatt.de/dae/owa/suchestellen.home).

REGISTRABLE QUALIFICATIONS FOR GERMAN DOCTORS GOING ABROAD

The registrable qualification granted in Germany is the *Zeugnis über die ärztliche Staatsprüfung* (State examination certificate in medicine), awarded by the competent authorities, and the *Zeugnis über die Vorbereitungszeit als Medizinalassistent* (certificate stating that the preparatory period as medical assistant has been completed).

For doctors who completed training in the former East Germany, the registrable qualification is the *Zeugnis über die ärztliche Staatsprüfung* (State examination certificate in medicine), awarded by the competent authorities after 30 June 1988. This must be accompanied by the certificate attesting to the practice of medicine during a period of practical training (*Arzt im Praktikum*). There are 37 universities with a faculty of medicine in Germany. The following are examples of licensing bodies (faculties of medicine) and the qualifications awarded:

- Freie Universität Berlin: *State Exam Med Berlin*
- Medizinische Hochschule Hannover: *State Exam Med Hannover*
- Ludwig-Maximilians Universität München: *State Exam Med München.*

Further information for medical students or research workers can be obtained from:

German Academic Exchange Service (DAAD)
34 Belgrave Square

London SW1X 8BQ
Tel: 0171 235 1736
Fax: 0171 235 9602
E-mail: info@daad.org.uk

DAAD offers scholarships for study and research in Germany and a number of information booklets are available from the above address.

There are IELTS centres and administrators (see p. 206) at the following addresses:

UCLES
Gierkrzeile 29
D-10585 Berlin
Tel: 00 49 (0)303 420 909
Fax: 00 49 (0)303 427 385

British Council
Hahnenstrasse 6
D-50667 Köln 1
Tel: 00 49 (0)221 206 4416
Fax: 00 49 (0)221 206 4455

Greece

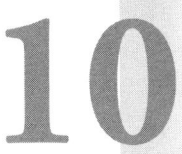

Joined EU: 1981
Area: 132 000 km²
Population (1998): 10.66 million
Population density: 81 persons / km²
Language: Greek
Currency: Drachma
Religion: Greek Orthodox (98%)
Government: Parliamentary republic
GDP per head (1994): 10 561 US$
Social security expenditure as % of GDP (1993): 15.5%
Health expenditure as % of GDP (1995): 5.8%
Infant mortality rate (1998): 7.26 deaths per 1000 live births
Average life expectancy at birth (1998): 75.8 (men); 81 (women); total 78.3 years
Unemployment (1997): 10%
Doctors per 10 000 population (1994): 38.8
Beds per 10 000 population (1994): 5.0

BACKGROUND

Greece is the eastern most of the southern EU states and the pace of life is somewhat adapted to the climate. Wages are low but so is the cost of living. Working hours allow for an afternoon siesta and trying to conduct administrative tasks can be frustrating. Having a decent grasp of Greek is mandatory, not simply for finding a job and organizing registration but also because a formal assessment of language needs to be undergone by EC doctors wishing to work in the Greek national health service.

The standard of medical training is generally considered lower than that of member states in northern Europe and obtaining recognition for posts worked in Greece as part of overall specialty training is difficult at present. Given the climate and the lifestyle, history and people, though, you may well not care.

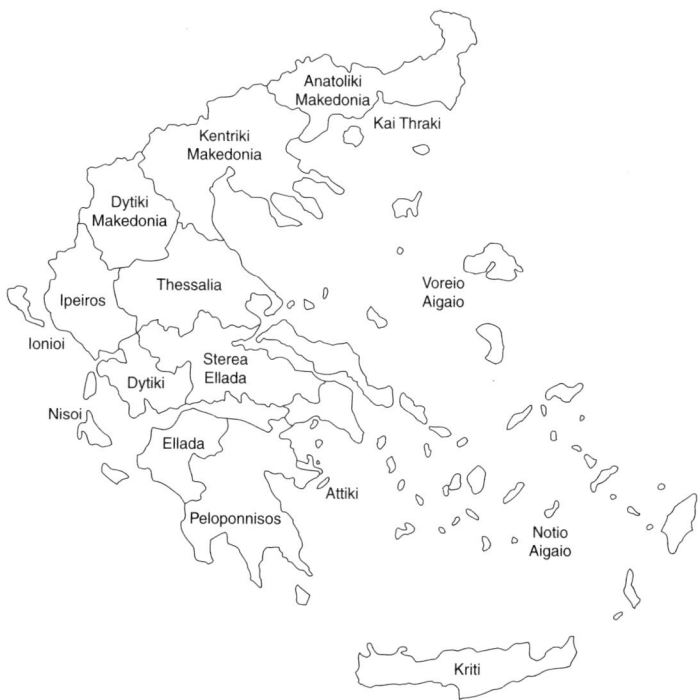

Fig. 10.1 Map of Greece.

The country is a parliamentary democracy. The single chamber parliament is elected by proportional representation. The present economic profile with its high inflation has prevented Greece from joining the single European currency. Developments are taking place in other areas, however, particularly transport infrastructure, as the country prepares to host the Olympic Games in 2004.

One-third of the total population of Greece lives in the Greater Athens area and most of the hospital-based medicine is centred in Athens and Salonika. As well as the mainland, there are over 2000 Greek islands, of which over 150 are inhabited. Island inhabitants make up over one fifth of the total population. In the past, these rural areas had rather sparse medical services but improvements in primary health care, together with compulsory periods of clinical service in rural hospitals as part of general training, have improved matters.

It is necessary to register with the police within eight days of arrival (or at the Aliens' Department Office, if staying in Athens). A residence permit is required for stays longer than three months although this can be difficult to obtain without first having proof of employment.

For accommodation, it is worth enquiring at one's place of employment. It is often difficult to find and is usually unfurnished; open contracts tend to be for periods of around 2 years.

Education is free from nursery to university level. It is compulsory from age 6 to 15 years.

LANGUAGE

Modern Greek began to evolve around the ninth century but did not become the official language of Greece until the nineteenth. The Greek alphabet dates from around 1000 B.C..

Greek is one language with which doctors will have a slight head start. Prefixes such as auto-, hetero- and micro-, and suffixes such as -meter, -phobia and -scope appear in everyday parlance as well as on the hospital shop floor.

As well as spoken Greek, known as Demotic, a derivative of Classical Greek known as Pure Greek may be encountered, having been revived for use in literature.

ORGANIZATION OF THE HEALTH SYSTEM

The Greek National Health Service was established in 1983 in an effort to curtail the growth of the private sector and to remove social inequalities of access to health care. The Ministry of Health was established at this time, by bringing together the health departments of the other ministries. Health policy is developed on a national level by the Ministry of Health and services in the private sector also come under its scrutiny. The population has compulsory insurance, but after that all medical care in the public sector is provided free.

The health service became decentralized as part of the 1983 reforms. In 1987, Greece was divided for administrative purposes into health districts (51 prefectures or *nomoi* and one autonomous region, Ayion Oros). The country is also divided into a smaller number of regions, or *diamerismata*, as shown on the map. Health-care needs at local level are assessed by Regional Health Departments, who in turn advise the government. Regional Health Departments were set up to serve as a link between the local populations and the government, although in practice they are sometimes understaffed and lack the necessary resources to function as they should.

Private practice was initially limited by these reforms and clinicians working full-time in public hospitals were not allowed to practise privately. New legislation was passed in 1991, however, encouraging the shift of health policy towards a more market-orientated approach. Private hospitals were allowed to be established and supplementation of services by private health care has been encouraged since.

Health insurance

The present social security system has been in existence for over 60 years and is based on obligatory insurance coverage. As well as health care, the system provides benefits including pensions and long-term disability payments. There are over 300 insurance funds, of which 80 cover sickness, the rest providing pensions and welfare coverage. The two largest insurance funds are the Social Security Fund (IKA in Greek), which covers more than 4 million industrial workers and clerical staff, and the Agricultural Workers' Fund (OGA in Greek), which covers more than 3 million farmers.

For health care the insurance funds provide their members with free hospital care and outpatient services within the public sector. Certain other non-emergency public sector services must be paid for and co-payments are charged for prescriptions (25% of the cost), except in the case of chronically ill patients. Patients attending at outpatient clinics without referral by the doctor attached to their insurance organization must also pay a fee.

In addition to the obligatory governmental insurance organizations, patients can obtain private insurance and this is becoming an increasing trend, as the provision of public health services does not always meet consumer expectation. For admission to a private hospital, the government insurance organization reimburses the amount that would be paid to public hospitals and the balance is met by the consumer.

Finance

Hospital care within the NHS is financed by the various insurance organizations and the state budget. The greater part of the cost is met by the latter, as fees set by the Ministry of Health for hospitalization and medical treatment represent only around 10% of the real cost. This proportion is reimbursed through insurance coverage, the remaining amount being financed by the state budget. Restructuring is presently under way with the aim of changing insurance reimbursement to reflect real cost more closely.

Hospital types

Within the NHS, hospitals are classified into regional general hospitals, which serve a population of between 1 000 000 and 1 500 000, and *district* general hospitals, which serve a population of between 50 000 and 500 000. Both types provide outpatient and accident and emergency services. The standard of care varies from hospital to hospital. Since the government lifted the restrictions on private practice, this sector provides hospital and ambulant care for an increasing number of patients.

Hospital management

Hospitals are managed by a hospital executive board, of which the president and majority of the staff are appointed by the Ministry of Health. The rest of the board comprises hospital workers and medical staff. Training in the field of management is somewhat underdeveloped compared to other countries and certain Greek hospitals are not run in the most efficient way.

Access to specialist care

Specialist services are available in the outpatient department of government hospitals. Patients are permitted to attend these clinics but if they do so without referral from the doctor of their insurance organization, they must pay a fee.

TRAINING AND TYPES OF POST

Undergraduate training is of 6 years' duration. Post-graduate training is for 5–7 years, depending on specialty. During this time, there is no formal assessment but trainees must sit a final examination before specialist status can be awarded.

The number of doctors has increased markedly over the past 30 years, so that the overall ratio of doctors to inhabitants is one of the highest in the EU. The distribution of doctors is uneven, with considerable clustering in Greater Athens and Salonika and few doctors in the more rural areas. Since the health-care reforms, attempts have been made to address this imbalance. There has been a greater focus on primary care, with improvement of local health centres, and training for hospital doctors now includes a compulsory practice attachment in a rural area.

Greece has also introduced a *numerus clausus* to reduce the number of students in medicine although it will take some years before any impact is made on the number of practising doctors. A large number of Greek-trained doctors come to Britain after qualifying. Greek nationals are the second-largest group of non-British EU nationals to be awarded British GMC full registration (see Fig. 18.2 p. 198).

PRACTICAL POINTS

Insurance and pensions

All NHS or self-employed doctors have to pay contributions to an insurance scheme. NHS doctors receive their principal pension from the Public Fund. Doctors are increasingly taking out supplementary private insurance.

Medical defence and professional disciplinary procedures

Personal medical indemnity is not obligatory in Greece. A new scheme for such defence is being set up but it is worth checking with the defence organization in one's native country to establish whether cover is provided for clinical practice in Greece.

Nursing

In the hospital setting, the standard of nursing is lower than in other EU states. Fewer than 35% of hospital nurses are fully qualified. The majority of nurses on the wards are care assistants, with a low level of general education and no formal nursing training.

REGISTRATION

The competent authority is the Panhellenic Medical Association. Applications for registration must be sent to this association, which then forwards the documents to the Ministry of Health. The latter then provides the licence to practise medicine in Greece and this is published in the *Official Gazette*.

All doctors have to be members of the national Panhellenic Medical Association and the local medical associations. There is an annual membership fee for both the national and local medical associations of around 3 000 and 8 000 drachma respectively.

Documents required for registration and a licence include the following:

- medical diploma
- documents regarding specialty status (if applicable)
- certificate of good standing (available from the GMC or equivalent competent authority)
- proof of good character (available from the British Embassy in Athens)
- proof of lack of juridical proceedings for physical or mental health reasons
- certificate of nationality (identity card/passport).

These must be sent to the Panhellenic Medical Association, together with an application form.

In order to be eligible for delivery of services, one must then register with the *local* medical association, submitting the following documents:

- license to practise medicine (see above)
- certificate of practice of medicine from EC country of origin (GMC certificate for UK nationals)
- certificates of diplomas.

Language testing is not required before acquiring the licence to practice but is mandatory for doctors from EU countries wishing to work in the Greek NHS.

FINDING A POST

Posts are advertised by the Ministry of Health or by insurance funds, and vacancies are also posted in daily newspapers and in the journal of the Panhellenic Medical Association and other medical journals (e.g. *IATPIKOΣ TYΠOΣ*). If applying from outside Greece, it is best to contact the Panhellenic Medical Association or one of the university teaching hospitals directly, to find out when posts are likely to be available (see 'List of hospitals', below).

LIST OF HOSPITALS

A full list of hospitals in Athens, as well as those in Salonika, is available from the Greek Embassy in London.

Aiginitio
B. Sofias 72
Tel: 00 30 (0)1 772 0811

Alexandra
B. Sofias 80
Tel: 00 30 (0)1 777 0431

Aretaio
E. Venizelou 76
Tel: 00 30 (0)1 723 8511

Ippokratio
B. Sofias 114
Tel: 00 30 (0)1 748 3770

Laïko
Ag. Thoma 17
Tel: 00 30 (0)1 777 1101

ADDRESSES

Competent authority
Panhellenic Medical Association
Ploutarchou 3
106 75 Athens
Tel: 00 30 (0)1 725 8660/61/62; 00 30 (0)1 381 6404/770 3733/ 777 4327
Fax: 00 30 (0)1 725 8663; 00 30 (0)1 384 1234

Greek Association of General Practitioners
N. Kountourioti 21, 5th Floor
546 25 Thessaloniki
Tel: 00 30 (0)31 539 995
Fax: 00 30 (0)31 550 048

REGISTRABLE QUALIFICATIONS FOR GREEK DOCTORS GOING ABROAD

The registrable qualification granted in Greece is the *Ptychio Iatrikes* (degree in medicine), awarded either by the faculty of medicine of a university or by the faculty of health sciences, department of medicine, of a university.

There are six faculties of medicine in Greece. Of these, Athens and Salonika are the largest. A list of the licensing bodies (faculties of medicine) and the qualifications awarded is shown below:

- National Capodistrian University of Athens: *Ptychio Iatrikes Athens*
- University of Crete: *Ptychio Iatrikes Crete*
- University of Ioannina: *Ptychio Iatrikes Ioannina*
- University of Patras: *Ptychio Iatrikes Patras*
- Aristotelian University of Thessaloniki: *Ptychio Iatrikes Thessalonika*
- University of Thrace: *Ptychio Iatrikes Thrace*.

There are IELTS centres and administrators (see p. 206) at the following addresses:

British Council
Examinations Section
17 Kolanaki Sq
PO Box 3488
GR-102 10 Athens
Tel: 00 30 (0)1 363 3211
Fax: 00 30 (0)1 363 4769

British Council
Ethnikis Amynis 9 (and Tsimiski Corner)
PO Box 50007
GR-540 13 Thessaloniki
Tel: 00 30 (0)31 235 236
Fax: 00 30 (0)31 282 498

For further information, particularly for medical students, contact:

Greek Cultural Institute
1a Holland Park
London W11 3TP
Tel: 0171 229 3850

Republic of Ireland (Eire)

11

Joined EU: 1973
Area: 70 280 km²
Population (1998): 3.62 million
Population density: 52 persons/km²
Languages: Irish; English
Currency: Punt
Religion: (93%) Roman Catholic
Government: Republic
GDP per head (1994): 14 171 US$
Social security expenditure as % of GDP (1993): 20.4%
Health expenditure as % of GDP (1995): 6.4%
Infant mortality rate (1998): 6.04 deaths per 1000 live births
Average life expectancy at birth (1998): 73.4 (men); 79.1 (women); total 76.2 years
Unemployment (1995): 11.8%
Doctors per 10 000 population (1995): 17.2
Beds per 10 000 population (1995): 5.0

BACKGROUND

The Republic of Ireland is a parliamentary democracy with a written constitution. There is a President, whose position as Head of State is chiefly apolitical, and a Prime Minister.

Ireland is presently Western Europe's fastest-growing economy, thanks largely to a decade of determined government effort, including reassessment of public finances, labour agreements and heavy investment in education and infrastructure. A large proportion of the economy is based on agriculture.

Rates of income tax and employees' national insurance contributions are high owing to the small workforce (unemployment is high). Inflation is low and rent, even in the capital city, Dublin, is relatively low.

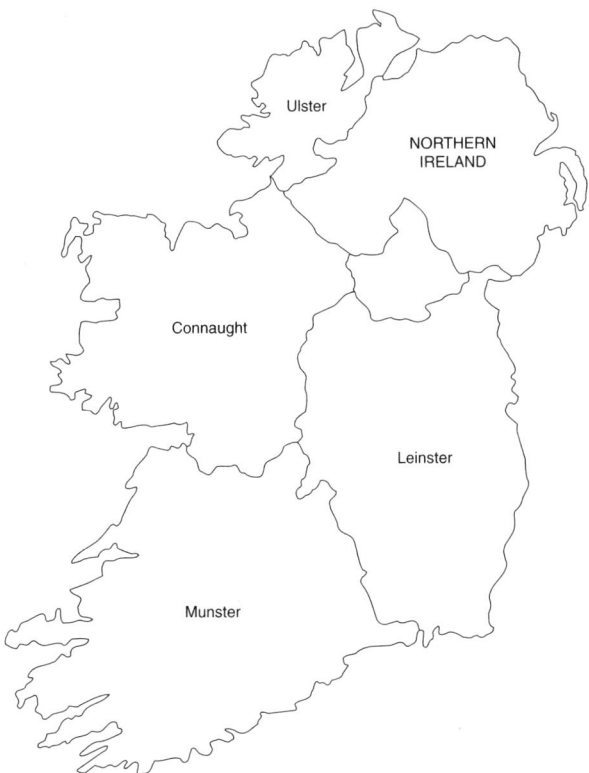

Fig. 11.1 Map of Northern Ireland and the Republic of Ireland.

Education is from a minimum age of 4 years (to start age 6 years at the latest) to a minimum age of 15 years.

LANGUAGE

Irish Gaelic, or Irish, is spoken by around one third of the population (1 million people) and is the official language of the Republic of Ireland together with English.

ORGANIZATION OF THE HEALTH SYSTEM

Policies on health care are made by the Department of Health, which was established as a separate department in 1947. Health-service provision, according to policy guidelines, is then dealt with by each of the eight local health boards.

The population served by a health board varies according to region, from around 200 000 to 1 230 000. The health board is made up of members of the county council (the majority), and those of the health professions. Some members are appointed by the Minister of Health.

Ireland has a number of authorities and boards which deal with specific aspects of the health system. A few are described in Box 11.1.

BOX 11.1
Irish health authorities and boards

National Drugs Advisory Board
- Set up by the Ministry of Health; works to monitor new products, check safety and collect and provide information concerning side-effects and precautions

Hospitals Council (Comhairle na nOspideal)
- Established under the Health Act in 1970. Members of the Council are appointed by the Ministry of Health and at least half of them must be consultants, the remainder representing nurses and administrators.
- Regulates the number and type of consultant appointments in hospitals which provide services under the Health Act and specifies qualifications for these appointments.
- Has an important advisory role in the development of hospital services

Voluntary Health Insurance Board
- Operates a state-sponsored scheme of health insurance to complement public health services; a non-profit-making statutory corporation of five members appointed by the Minister of Health

Medical Registration Council
- A statutory corporation in charge of registration of medical practitioners. Comprises 11 members, including 2 government nominees, 2 members elected by medical practitioners and nominees of medical schools

Health Research Board
- A national body appointed by the Ministry of Health in charge of organizing and carrying out research in medicine and the health services

---

Finance

Health-care services are provided largely by the public agencies and funded by the Exchequer. Funding is primarily from general taxation. Certain services are paid in full or in part, depending on different income groups. These payments are sustained in part by a monopoly State-sponsored Voluntary Health Insurance Board, operating on what are known as 'community rating' principles. Some services are also provided by voluntary agencies on behalf on health boards.

There is also a small private sector, which operates independently from the public health-care system. Some private spending is supported, indirectly, from public funds through tax relief on health insurance premia. Other minor sources of health service funding include:

- a small contribution of earmarked health tax, collected under the general taxation system
- fundraising by voluntary groups and patients' support associations
- funds provided from the proceeds of a national lottery
- receipts under EC Regulations related to the treatment in Ireland of nationals of other member states.

Hospital types

There are three broad categories, as follows:

1. *Voluntary* (not-for-profit) hospitals, which are owned and operated by religious orders or function under the management of boards appointed by the Minister for Health. Almost all income for these hospitals comes directly from the Department of Health as an annual allowance. Most of these hospitals are located in the larger population centres, predominantly Dublin. Due to their location, they provide most of the higher-level specialties and account for around half of acute medical beds.

2. *Health Board* hospitals are owned, managed and funded by the local health boards. The health boards receive an annual allowance from the Department of Health and are then responsible for allocating the available funds between the hospitals within the geographical area.

3. *Private* hospitals are owned and managed by private organizations and, in general, receive no direct funding from the State. They make up a small percentage of hospital services.

Over the past few years, hospital services have been rationalized, with expensive equipment and skilled staff being concentrated in large units and with promotion of outpatient and day-care services.

Access to specialist care

There are two categories of eligibility for health services:

- *Category 1* refers to members of the community who cannot afford medical services for themselves or their dependants, according to criteria outlined by the Chief Executive Officer of the local health board. People in this category are issued with a medical card and receive a broad range of services free of charge — namely, general practitioner services and inpatient and outpatient hospital services in public wards.

- *Category 2* individuals are those with limited eligibility for state health service provision. They are entitled to all inpatient and outpatient services, subject to certain charges.

Defects discovered at school health and child developmental examinations are treated free in public hospital wards, irrespective of the income of the parents, as are patients injured in road traffic accidents. Certain other services may be provided free of charge in special circumstances, according to the discretion of the Chief Executive Officers of health boards.

GPs practise gatekeeping, whereby all patients must be assessed first before being considered for specialist referral.

TRAINING AND TYPES OF POST

Working hours and grades of hospital doctor are similar to the United Kingdom system. There are five medical schools in Ireland, of which four are public. Undergraduate studies are of 6 years' duration, divided into pre-clinical and clinical modules. After qualifying, all doctors must work for 1 year (6 months in medicine and 6 months in surgery) as a junior house officer or *intern*. At the end of this year, provided the house officer has worked to a satisfactory standard, he or she is awarded full registration with the national competent authority and is then eligible for a senior house officer (SHO) post. Posts as an SHO are generally for periods of between 6 months and 2 years. During this period, the SHO has the opportunity to consider future specialization and must sit an examination to obtain Membership of the appropriate Royal College (see 'Addresses', below).

Once this has been obtained the next grade up is specialist registrar. The old grading system of registrar and senior registrar is in the process of being disbanded and eventually, the title 'specialist registrar' will cover all doctors between SHO and consultant level.

REGISTRATION

Work permits are not required for members of EU member states but all doctors must be registered with the national competent authority, the Irish Medical Council. Documents required for registration vary according to nationality and country of basic medical training. In general, the following information is required and must be forwarded to the Registrar at the Medical Council:

- the name of the medical school affiliated to the university from which the primary degree/diploma was obtained
- the name of the university to which the medical school is affiliated

- the exact date the degree / diploma was conferred
- the applicant's nationality.

On receipt of this, the Medical Council can then write with further information regarding the documents necessary for registration. For EU nationals, this generally includes the following:

- curriculum vitae concerning medical career
- certificate of full registration with native competent authority
- certificate of good standing issued by native competent authority within 3 months of the application for registration with the Irish Medical Council
- passport or other certificate of nationality.

FINDING A POST

Posts are advertised in the journal of the Irish Medical Association and certain appointments are mentioned in the classified section of the *British Medical Journal*. It is also worth contacting the medical staffing department of the relevant hospital in order to find out when suitable posts are likely to be advertised.

LIST OF HOSPITALS

The main teaching hospitals attached to faculties of medicine are listed here for each university town. A complete list of hospitals is available from the Department of Health and the Voluntary Health Insurance Board, for public and private hospitals, respectively.

St James's Hospital
1 James Street
Dublin 8
Tel: 00 353 (0)1 453 7941

Beaumont Hospital
9 Beaumont Road
Dublin 9
Tel: 00 353 (0)1 837 7755

Our Lady's Hospital for Sick Children
Crumlin
Dublin 12
Tel: 00 353 (0)1 455 8111

Cork University Hospital
Wilton
Cork
Tel: 00 353 (0)2 190 3000

University College Hospital
Newcastle Road
Galway

ADDRESSES

Competent authority
Comhairle na nDochtúirí Leighis
Medical Council
Lynn House
Portobello Court
Lower Rathimines Road
Dublin 6
Tel: 00 353 (0)1 496 5588
Fax: 00 353 (0)1 496 5972

Irish Medical Organization
10 Fitzwilliam Place
Dublin 2
Tel: 00 353 (0)1 767 273
Fax: 00 353 (0)1 612 758

Royal College of Physicians of Ireland
6 Kildare Street
Dublin 2
Tel: 00 353 (0)1 661 6677

Royal College of Surgeons of Ireland
123 St Stephen's Green
Dublin 2
Tel: 00 353 (0)1 402 2261

Irish College of General Practitioners
Corrigan House
Fenian Street
Dublin 2
Tel: 00 353 (0)1 676 3705

Irish Medical News
Taney Hall

Eglington Terrace
Dublin 14

Department of Health
Hawkins House
Hawkins Street
Dublin 2

Voluntary Health Insurance Board
VHI House
20 Lower Abbey Street
Dublin 1
Tel: 00 353 (0)1 872 4499,
00 353 (0)1 874 9171

REGISTRABLE QUALIFICATIONS FOR IRISH DOCTORS GOING ABROAD

The registrable qualification granted in Ireland is the *primary qualification*, awarded after passing a qualifying examination held by a competent examining body, and a *Certificate of experience*, granted by that body, which gives entitlement to registration as a fully registered medical practitioner.

Ireland has universities in Dublin, Cork and Galway with faculties of medicine. The following is an example of two licensing bodies (faculties of medicine) and the qualifications awarded:

- University of Dublin: *MD BCh Dubl*
- National University of Ireland: *MB BCh NU Irel.*

Further information, particularly for medical students or research workers, is available from:

Higher Education Authority
21 Fitzwilliam Square
Dublin 2
Tel: 00 353 (0)1 661 2748

Italy

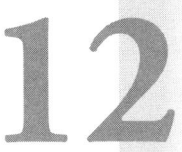

Joined EU: 1957
Area: 301 000 km²
Population (1998): 56.8 million
Population density: 189/persons/km²
Language: Italian
Currency: Lira
Religion: Roman Catholic (98%)
Government: Republic
GDP per head (1994): 17 086 US$
Social security expenditure as % of GDP (1993): 24.5%
Health expenditure as % of GDP (1995): 7.7%
Infant mortality rate (1998): 6.4 deaths per 1000 live births
Average life expectancy at birth (1998): 75.3 (men); 81.7 (women); total 78.4 years
Unemployment (1997): 12.2%
Doctors per 10 000 population (1992): 16.5
Beds per 10 000 population (1994): 6.5

BACKGROUND

Italy is a parliamentary democracy. The government is based in Rome, the capital city, but the commercial and industrial centre is Milan. The country has a north–south divide comparable to that in Britain. The northern regions, particularly Lombardy, Piedmont and Liguria, are highly industrialized and contain around half the total population, while the south is underdeveloped and poor. Although Italy's economy has grown in recent years, it has also hit recession and unemployment is high.

There is no need to enthuse about the art, history, music, language, food and people of this beautiful country and the space allotted here would do them no justice. The practical aspects of living in Italy, in contrast, can prove

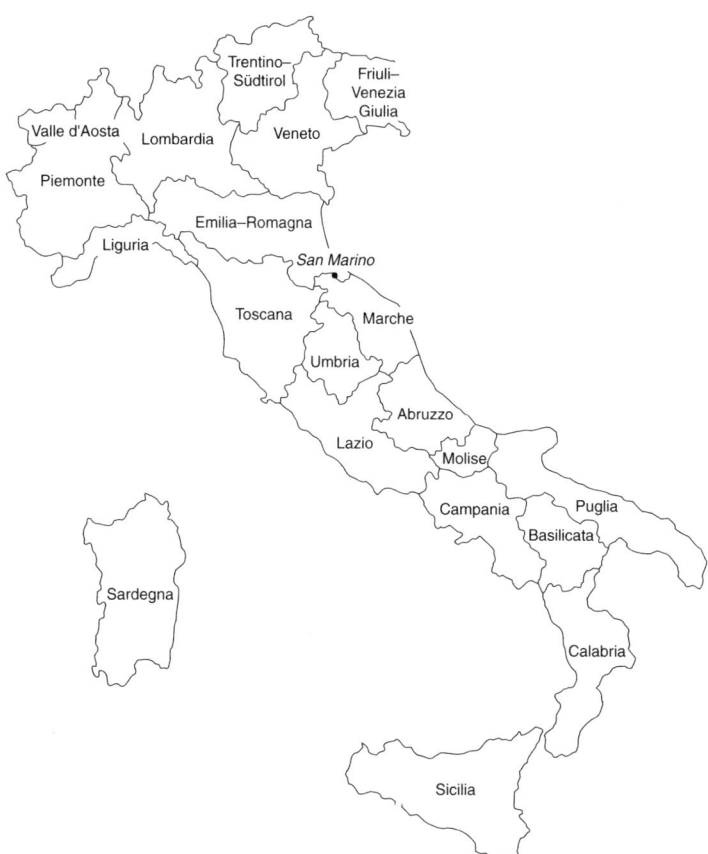

Fig. 12.1 Map of Italy.

to be less appealing. Dealing with administrative bodies can be a slow and frustrating process and medical standards are not always those enjoyed by doctors practising further north.

EU nationals who wish to stay in Italy must register with the local police within 7 days of arrival. They must also obtain a tax number, as this is required when registering a car, buying a flat or finding a job. As well as income tax, there is a local tax which includes a property tax.

The cost of living is generally lower than in most northern European countries but is high in cities, particularly Rome and Venice. Hospital doctors' salaries are also correspondingly lower. At present, underemployment and unemployment amongst medical professionals are high.

School is compulsory from age 5 years. School-leavers wishing to attend university must complete a total of 13 years at school (5 years' primary, 3 years' lower secondary and 5 years' secondary) and take the national diploma, the *maturità*.

LANGUAGE

Italian is a member of the Romance family of languages. As well as being the national language of Italy, it is one of the four official languages of Switzerland. In common with other languages described in this book, Italian has several dialects which differ considerably from the 'textbook' Italian learned in schools. The alphabet consists of 21 letters, j, k, w, x and y appearing only in foreign (non-Italian) words.

Although Italian is the official language, there are a number of non-Italian-speaking minorities; German is also used officially in the Trentino–Alto Adige region (see chapter 9) and there are Slavs in the Trieste area.

Rhaeto-Romanic is a collective term for three dialects of the Romance family spoken in north-eastern Italy and south-eastern Switzerland. Around 90% of the more than 500 000 speakers live in Italy although, unlike in Switzerland, the dialects have no official status there. The two Rhaeto-Romanic dialects of Italy are Friulian, with around 500 000 speakers in the region of Friuli, near the border with Austria and Slovenia, and Ladin, with around 10 000 speakers in Alto Adige to the west. The continued survival of these dialects is largely due to the geographical isolation of the people, as these areas are rural and mountainous.

ORGANIZATION OF THE HEALTH SYSTEM

Italy's national health-care system was established in December 1978, with the passing of the Health-Care Reform Act. This Act set out guidelines allowing a previously disorganized and divided system to develop a more unified structure. Whereas prior to the Act health-care provision had been based on sickness benefit funds, the new health system is now free of charge and cover is provided for the whole of the employed working population, including registered foreigners. Services within the national health-care system are comprehensive, including prevention, treatment and rehabilitation, and are uniform nationwide.

The national health-care service is organized at central, regional and local levels. At central level, the State establishes principles for planning, policy-making and financing. There is an operational body (the Ministry of Health) and four technical consultative bodies (the National Health Council, the Superior Institute for Industrial Safety and Prevention, the Superior Health

Council and the Superior Institute of Health). Funds from the state budget are assigned to the regions, which in turn allocate the resources to the *local health units*. The latter form the basis of the entire health-care system (see below). Organizations functioning privately work under a convention with the State.

As well as dealing with resource allocation, the regions are responsible for supervising planning and setting standards of care and this is done according to national guidelines. The regional bodies also pass legislation applying to hospital and general health care. This covers the areas listed in Box 12.1.

BOX 12.1
Areas covered by regional legislation

- Implementation of state regulations and guidelines
- Prevention and treatment of infectious diseases
- Control of toxic or hazardous products, including X-ray equipment
- Control of dietetic products, baby food and cosmetics.

Local health units provide health care at municipal level. These units are dependent on the region for planning, financing and regulation of personnel but have considerable autonomy and play a key role in the health-care system. They have responsibilities within a specific geographic area which are not already defined at state or regional level. Since the Act, the national obligation to provide hospitals has been transferred to the local health units and hospital management is assigned directly to the unit management arm.

Hospitals outside the National Health Service are managed independently and care provided in military hospitals is dealt with by the State.

Finance

The health service is funded by the government and by direct contributions from employees and employers. Funds for hospital care come from the state budget, whether this care is provided in public organizations or in private organizations working under a convention with the State. The self-employed pay a *health tax*. Private or company-based insurance is supplementary.

GP and outpatient consultations within the national health-care service are free. For inpatient care, there are co-payments, which are paid for *per diem*. Prescriptions have a fixed charge, although there are a number of exceptions for certain drugs or medical conditions. Pharmaceutical services are provided by private pharmacies adhering to a specific national convention.

Hospital types

Military hospitals aside, hospitals are divided into:

- public hospitals belonging to the local health units
- teaching hospitals linked to a university
- private hospitals belonging to religious orders.

Hospital care within the national health sector is provided in the first two. Due to unified health-care provision, private agencies must be considered distributors of public services, although they are able to retain private legal status.

Two hospitals, Galliera Hospital in Genoa and Mauriziano Hospital in Turin, are autonomous and have special legal status. Most hospitals are multi- rather than single-specialty, with university hospitals providing the bulk of tertiary care. Psychiatric services are integrated into the general health care provided by public hospitals.

Access to specialist care

Patients can choose their own GP but must register within their area. In practice, the choice is restricted, as GPs are allowed a maximum of 1500 patients on their lists. The Italian health service runs a gatekeeper system for access to specialist care, so that hospital and outpatient specialist care require GP referral. In the hospital setting, some specialists provide primary care and paediatricians provide primary care for children up to the age of 12 years.

TRAINING AND TYPES OF POST

As mentioned, there is considerable unemployment and underemployment amongst medical professionals in Italy; this situation is unlikely to improve, as medical student intake continues to be high. There was a recent attempt to reduce student numbers by introducing a *numerus clausus*. Unfortunately, a number of students who had been rejected took the universities to court and ended up winning their appeal and so it is difficult to anticipate how effective such control measures are likely to be.

Undergraduate studies are of 6 years' duration. A large part of training is university- rather than hospital-based and even clinical skills are taught in the lecture theatre rather than at the bedside.

In the hospital setting, doctors in training were previously stratified at three levels: *assistenti* (junior staff), *aluti* (senior staff) and a *primario* (unit head). The hierarchy has now been reduced to two levels and conditions of employment have been changed. The unit head is *di secondo livello* and is now no longer offered a lifelong contract but rather a 5-year position, which can be renewable if 'predetermined goals' are fulfilled. All staff more junior to the unit head are *di primo livello*. This new nomenclature implies universal equality, although clearly some staff will be more 'equal' than others, depending on experience post-qualification.

Italy does not have a large, cohesive doctors' union. Most hospital doctors join one of the various political trade unions or one of a multitude of doctor-only guilds. Hospital clinicians working full-time have an exclusive contract with health-care agencies and are therefore not allowed to engage in private practice. Hospital doctors with part-time contracts are permitted to practise privately — that is, those salaried for 75% commitment or less to the NHS. GPs are paid on a capitation system, with negotiated fees for particular services.

PRACTICAL POINTS

Waiting lists points

Although health care is provided free of charge, there are waiting lists for a number of specialist services and many Italian patients seek treatment abroad, particularly in France, where waiting lists are shorter.

REGISTRATION

Registration in Italy is slow and great patience plus a reasonable knowledge of Italian are required. Diploma requirements for registration vary, depending on original country of qualification; more information can be obtained from the competent authority (see 'Addresses', below). (It is best to either telephone or write, as faxing can be unreliable.) The competent authority also issues a registration application form which needs to be completed and returned with the necessary documents. Registration is dealt with at regional level and so one needs to have an idea of which part of the country employment is likely to be based in.

FINDING A POST

The competent authority has some information regarding available posts although, with the considerable unemployment and underemployment in Italy, it may be more rewarding to contact the relevant department of one of the main teaching hospitals directly.

LIST OF HOSPITALS

A list is available from the competent authority (see below).

ADDRESSES

Competent authority (*Registering body and main professional association*)
Federazione Nazionale degli Ordini dei Medici (FNOOMM)
Piazza Cola di Rienzo 80/A
00192 Roma
Tel: 00 39(0)6 687 40 34
Fax: 00 39(0)6 687 67 39

SIMG (*Society of Italian General Practice*)
Via il Prato 60
50123 Firenze
Tel: 00 39(0)55 28 40 30

REGISTRABLE QUALIFICATIONS FOR ITALIAN DOCTORS GOING ABROAD

The registrable qualification granted in Italy is the *Diploma di laurea in medicina e chirurgia* (Diploma of graduate in medicine and surgery), awarded by a university, accompanied by the *Diploma di abilitazione all'esercizio della medicina e chirurgia* (diploma confirming the right to practise medicine and surgery), awarded by the State Examining Commission.

There are over 30 universities with faculties of medicine in Italy, of which three are in Rome. The following are examples of licensing bodies (faculties of medicine) and the qualifications awarded:

- Università di Firenze: *State DMS Florence*
- Università di Milano: *State DMS Milan*
- Università di Roma Tor Vergata: *State DMS Rome Tor Vergata.*

For further information, the following is a useful source:

Italian Cultural Institute
39 Belgrave Square
London SW1X 8NX
Tel: 0171 235 1461

Luxembourg

Joined EU: 1957
Area: 2580/km²
Population (1998): 0.43 million
Population density: 167 persons / km²
Languages: Luxembourgish; French; German
Currency: Luxembourg franc
Religion: Roman Catholic (97%)
Government: Constitutional monarchy
GDP per head (1994): 26 979 US$
Social security expenditure as % of GDP (1993): 24.0%
Health expenditure as % of GDP (1995): 7.0%
Infant mortality rate (1998): 5.04 deaths per 1000 live births
Average life expectancy at birth (1998): 74.4 (men); 80.7 (women); total 77.5 years
Unemployment (1997): 3.5%
Doctors per 10 000 population (1993): 22.3
Beds per 10 000 population (1994): 11.1

BACKGROUND

Do not be misled by the diminutive size of the Grand Duchy of Luxembourg. Although children grow up to be trilingual, the national language is Luxembourgish or more correctly Letzebuergesch, and the population has a strong sense of national identity. French is the main language of the courts, German of the press.

Luxembourg is a representative democracy in the form of a constitutional hereditary monarchy. The Grand Duke is Head of State. The government is led by a Prime Minister and is usually formed by a coalition; the Chamber is elected every 5 years.

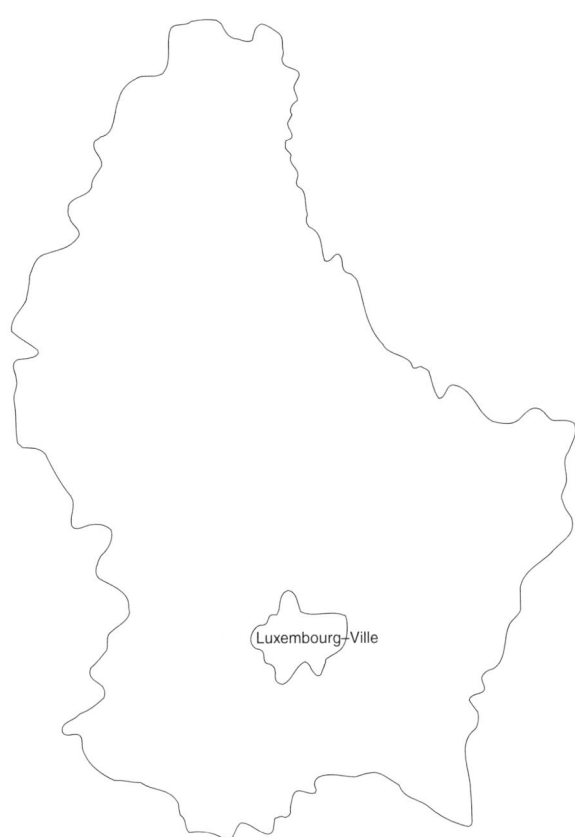

Fig. 13.1 Map of Luxembourg.

Luxembourg is bitterly cold in winter, particularly in the higher altitudes of the Ardennes region, but green and lush in summer. The Grand Duchy is divided into three districts (Luxembourg, Diekirch and Grevenmacher), 12 *cantons* and 118 municipalities. (For further information regarding national statistics, Luxembourg has its own website at www.statec.lu.)

The standard of living is Luxembourg is generally high, and inflation and unemployment are low. Tax-payers are divided into those single or divorced, those widowed and those over 65 years. Married people are taxed jointly. As well as income tax, there are taxes on capital yields and property. There is no car registration tax. Medical facilities are of a high standard but costly, although social security reimburses most bills.

Schooling takes place in the national language from 4–5 years; French is introduced at the age of 5 and German from age 6.

LANGUAGE

Letzebuergesch is basically a Moselle-Frankish dialect of German (see Chapter 9) but is thought of as a separate language because Luxembourg is a separate country. There are around 350 000 speakers.

ORGANIZATION OF THE HEALTH SYSTEM

Health care in Luxembourg is based on a system of compulsory insurance, with contributions from public authorities. Insurance is paid to sick funds, which are organized on the basis of occupational groups. Contributions are paid in part by the insured person and in part by the employer. The various insurance schemes are grouped together to form the Union of Sickness Funds (*Union des Caisses de Maladie*). This creates uniformity between the schemes and encourages equity in the benefits provided. There is a collective agreement on health-service tariffs which is negotiated between the Union of Sickness Funds and the representatives of the service-providers (the national medical association). This agreement applies nationally to all medical practitioners.

Hospital planning, financing and accreditation is dealt with by the Ministry of Health. The Ministry also supervises medical and paramedical practitioners. The Social Security Minister is responsible for health and maternity insurance, old age pension, disability insurance and survivors' benefits, insurance for industrial injury and occupational disease, family allowances and unemployment benefit.

Finance

Within the insurance system, medical fees are paid by the sickness funds. For inpatient hospital treatment, charges are met directly by the sickness funds by a third-party system of payment. Other medical treatment in specialist outpatient or GP settings is paid for by the patient on a fee-for-service basis. Patients are then reimbursed by the sickness funds, the amount depending on social status and type of treatment received. ('Life-savers' are reimbursed at 100%.) Doctors in Luxembourg are not allowed to practice outside the social security system and so there are no individual private practices. Charges are fixed as described above. As well as insurance contributions, Luxembourg's health system is funded by contributions from public authorities.

Hospital types

Four types of health-care establishment are defined by law. These are shown in Box 13.1.

> **BOX 13.1**
> **Types of health-care establishment in Luxembourg**
> - Institutes for the acute phase of illness
> - Institutes intended for lengthy stays (medium or long-term)
> - Specialist institutes (psychiatry, oncology)
> - Diagnostic centres

Hospitals for acute medical care are divided into regional, general and local, according to size and level of specialization:

- *Regional* hospitals are the closest equivalent to a UK teaching hospital. They provide permanent duty and emergency services and serve a large geographical area.
- *General* hospitals serve a limited geographical area and provide only the major medical and surgical disciplines. They tend not to have a 24-hour acute admission service.
- *Local* hospitals provide medical services only.

Half the hospitals in Luxembourg are private and belong to religious communities or non-profit-making organizations. The rest are public, semi-public or run by local authorities. Private premises are financed by private institutions and sometimes by government grants.

Hospital management

Hospital management is the responsibility of a number of councils (namely, the Hospital Council, the Medical Council and the Hospital Authority of Luxembourg), whose members are nominated by the Health Minister. Any changes proposed by these councils must be approved by this Minister. For example, the distribution of hospital beds between the three regions (northern, central and southern) is laid down by law. Any change in bed numbers or transfer between services must be discussed at council level and cannot be implemented without ministerial approval.

Access to specialist care

There is no gatekeeper system in Luxembourg and patients are free to select any physician, any service-provider and any hospital they choose. A procedure exists called the *Belegartztsystem* whereby a physician is approved by a hospital and is assigned a number of hospital beds for patient treatment. The approved physician can then use these beds when he or she wishes to admit a patient by applying directly to the owner of the hospital.

TRAINING AND TYPES OF POST

There is no medical school in Luxembourg and so Luxembourg nationals must train elsewhere to obtain the primary medical diploma. Most go to France, Belgium or Germany, as French and German are the second and third languages taught in schools. Once the diploma is obtained, they must register at the national competent authority before they can practise in Luxembourg. (See 'Registration', below.)

PRACTICAL POINTS

Terms and conditions

Physicians are either salaried or paid on a fee-for-service basis, depending on type of employment. Those at the Centre Hospitalier de Luxembourg (Luxembourg Hospital Complex) are paid at a flat rate and their salaries are taken from the body of income generated by the hospital. For clinics, consultants are paid on a sessional basis. Approved physicians who use the *Belegarztsystem* are paid on a fee-for-service basis.

At the Centre Hospitalier de Luxembourg and the Princesse Marie-Astrid Hospital at Niederkorn, part-time and full-time physicians have contracts under private law.

Medical defence and professional disciplinary procedures

Although physicians are appointed and dismissed by the hospital boards of directors, the practice of medical and paramedical practitioners comes under the jurisdiction of the Ministry of Health. Insurance against professional liability is not obligatory, although it is considered an ethical obligation. The National Medical Association recommends that its members insure themselves against claims to the order of around Lfrs 50 million. Although there are no official language tests before registering (see 'Registration', below), a doctor needs sufficient knowledge of the national languages (Luxembourgish, French and German) to practise. If a doctor commits a fault in the exercise of his or her profession through insufficient linguistic understanding, he or she is fully responsible.

Insurance and pensions

Physicians employed by the State are paid according to the remuneration scheme for civil servants. The medical profession forms part of the group of independent professional workers and since 1964 has been affiliated to the obligatory superannuation fund of private employees. The premium is related to maximum and minimum levels of gross income. It provides for a pension for widows and orphans and entitlement to benefit in case of invalidity. All these elements are index-linked to the cost of living and, moreover, are regularly adjusted by the government. Further information is available from the *Caisse de Pension des Employés Privés* (see 'Addresses' below).

The National Medical Association has information concerning superannuation and other schemes such as income protection plans and critical illness cover. The medical profession may also join a voluntary burial fund recommended by the National Medical Association. Further information is available from the *Caisse de Mutuelle des Professions Libérales et Indépendantes* (see 'Addresses', below).

REGISTRATION

The primary qualification of all doctors practising in Luxembourg has been awarded elsewhere, as the country has no faculty of medicine. Doctors must still register with the competent authority, however, and this is done by obtaining an application form and returning it together with the documents listed by the authority (original medical diploma, certificate of nationality and certificate of good standing, issued by the native competent authority).

There is no formal language testing for EU nationals but Article 6 of the Law on the Medical Profession of October 1995 demands that the doctor has sufficient linguistic knowledge for the practice of the profession in Luxembourg.

No fees are payable for registration and, as all doctors must practise within the social security system, entry into it is automatic on registration.

FINDING A POST

The leading medical journal is *Le Corps médical*.

There is no need for the advertisement of vacancies since registered practitioners may set up practice wherever they wish. For hospital posts, the relevant hospital should be contacted directly.

LIST OF HOSPITALS

Centre Hospitalier de Luxembourg
4 rue Nicolas-Ernest Barble
Luxembourg
Tel: 00 352 (0)44 11–1

Hôpital Princesse Marie-Astrid
187 avenue de la Liberté
Differdange Tel: 00 352 (0)58 46 46–1

ADDRESSES

Competent authority
Association des Médecins et Médecins-Dentistes du Grand Duché de Luxembourg
29 rue de Vianden
2680 Luxembourg-Ville
Tel: 00 352 (0)44 40 33
Fax: 00 352 (0)45 83 49

National medical association
Le Corps Médical
c/o Association des Médecins, etc.
Address as above.

National Registration Health Authority
Ministère de la Santé
57 boulevard de la Pétrusse
2320 Luxembourg-Ville

National Social Security Health Authority
Ministère de la Sécurité Sociale
26 rue Zithe
2763 Luxembourg-Ville

Comité Central de l'Union des Caisses de Maladie
Address as for Ministère de la Sécurité Sociale, above

Doctors' Pension Fund and Sickness Insurance
Caisse de Pension des Employés Privés
IA boulevard Prince Henri
1724 Luxembourg-Ville

Caisse Mutuelle des Professions Libérales et Indépendantes
c/o Fiduciaire Portic SA
44 rue Schrobigen
2526 Luxembourg-Ville

REGISTRABLE QUALIFICATIONS FOR DOCTORS FROM LUXEMBOURG GOING ABROAD

The registrable qualification is the *Diplôme d'État de docteur en médecine*, *chirurgie et accouchements* (State diploma of doctor of medicine, surgery and obstetrics), awarded by the State Examining Board and endorsed by the Minister of Education, and the *Certificate de stage* (Certificate of practical training), endorsed by the Minister for Public Health.

The Grand Duchy of Luxembourg has no university with a faculty of medicine and Luxembourg nationals thus must train elsewhere to obtain a medical diploma. Once this diploma has been recognized by the national competent authority, the equivalent qualification is the *MD Luxembourg*.

Further information for medical students or research workers is available from:

Ministère de l'Éducation Nationale
29 rue Aldringen
L-2926 Luxembourg
Tel: 00 352 (0)478 5100

The Netherlands 14

Joined EU: 1957
Area: 41 500 km²
Population (1998): 15.73 million
Population density: 379 persons / km²
Language: Dutch
Currency: Guilder
Religion: Catholic (34%); Protestant (25%); unaffiliated (36%)
Government: Constitutional monarchy
GDP per head (1994): 17 317 US$
Social security expenditure as % of GDP (1993): 32.1%
Health expenditure as % of GDP (1995): 8.8%
Infant mortality rate (1998): 5.17 deaths per 1000 live births
Average life expectancy at birth (1998): 75.1 (men); 81 (women); total 78 years
Unemployment (1997): 6.9%
Doctors per 10 000 population (1993): 30.2
Beds per 10 000 population (1995): 11.3

BACKGROUND

The Netherlands is a constitutional monarchy with a two-chamber parliament. The Hague is the political and diplomatic centre, although the capital city is Amsterdam. The Head of Government is the Prime Minister and Queen Beatrice is the Head of State.

Almost a quarter of the territory is below sea level and was formed by land reclamation. The highest point is at Vaalserberg (Limburg), 321 metres (900 feet) above sea level.

The Dutch enjoy good living and are keen on outdoor pursuits. There is a very good rail system and easy access to other parts of Europe. They also have a well-developed system of cycle paths in and around town.

Social security payments are high but so are the benefits.

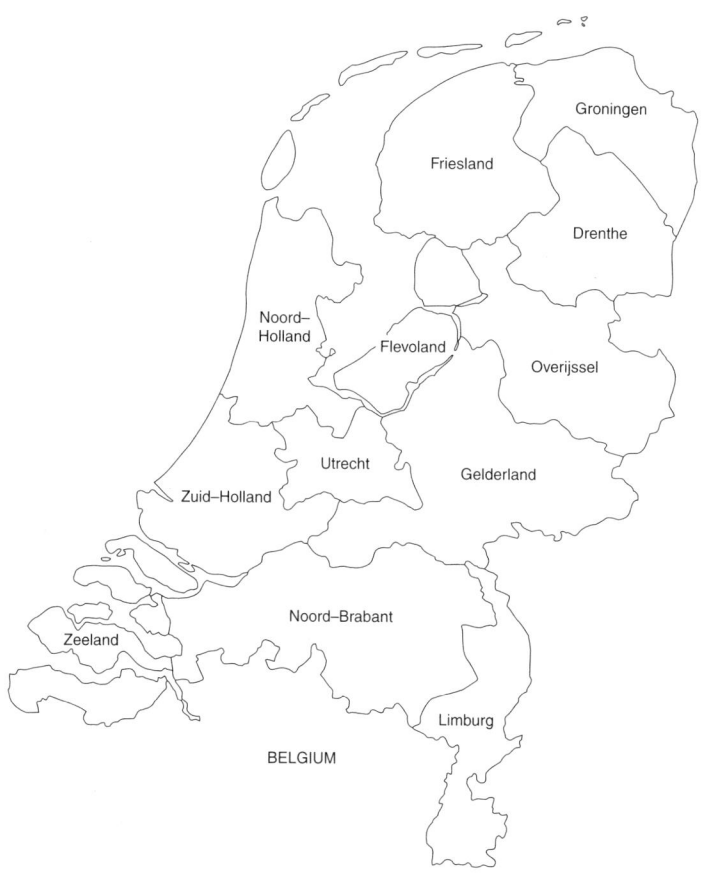

Fig. 14.1 Map of the Netherlands.

Education is free and compulsory from 5–16 years. In Dutch schools, English is taught from the age of 10 and lessons in a third language begin at the age of 12.

LANGUAGE

Dutch is a Germanic language like German and English. Although it is the closest to English of any of the major languages, the sentence structure follows that of German, with verbs placed at the end.

Frisian is spoken in the northern province of Friesland (capital Leeuwarden), which includes the outlying West Frisian Islands. There are around 300 000 speakers in this province, who are generally referred to as

West Frisians. The language is also spoken by about 10 000 other people in Germany in the northernmost province of Schleswig-Holstein which borders Denmark, and on the adjacent North Frisian Islands to the west. These people are known as North Frisians. Frisian is another Germanic language, close to English and Dutch.

ORGANIZATION OF THE HEALTH SYSTEM

Around 80% of hospitals and other services are private foundations or associations as opposed to being government-run.

Public health is the responsibility of the Minister of Welfare, Health and Cultural Affairs. The Minister is aided by five advisory bodies which deal with the various aspects of health care and services (see Box 14.1).

BOX 14.1
Advisory bodies in the Netherlands

- The *National Advisory Council for Public Health* is concerned with developments in health care and also deals with checking the qualifications of medical and paramedical practitioners.
- The *Health Council* advises on developments in medical science.
- The *Hospital Facilities Board* advises on the planning and building of hospitals according to the Health Facilities Act. There are national guidelines for drawing up provincial plans and a licence must be obtained from the Minister of Welfare, Health and Cultural Affairs before a health-care institution may be built.
- The *Health Insurance Funds Council* advises on the application of the Health Insurance Act and Exceptional Medical Expenses Compensation Act (AWBZ).
- The *Central Body for Health Care Charges* (COTG) advises on tariffs, fees and prices.

The various fields of planning, financing, insurance and tariffs for treatment are regulated by the central government. The Netherlands is divided into provinces and municipalities which have executive powers in health care. The municipalities decide upon how many general practitioners may establish practices. The number of clinical posts in hospitals is authorized by the Ministry of Welfare, Health and Cultural Affairs. The government is responsible for providing services which private institutions have not provided.

Health insurance

Dutch health care is based on a system of insurance schemes. A social insurance scheme or sick fund exists for people in employment and covers around two-thirds of the population. Those on higher incomes must take out private insurance but premiums are tax-deductible. Both sick funds and private insurance are administered by health insurance companies based in the different provinces. Those unable to afford insurance and the unemployed are covered by social security provisions. (See Box 14.2 for further details.)

BOX 14.2
Structure of insurance schemes in the Netherlands

There are three principal schemes:

1. *The Exceptional Medical Expenses Compensation Act (AWBZ)*. This is a compulsory scheme for everyone in the Netherlands, providing for so-called serious medical risks. Cover includes long stays in hospital, nursing homes, homes for the disabled and home nursing.
2. *Insurance for the cost of medical care (hospital and GP fees)*. This is dependent on income and employment status. The scheme is divided into health insurance funds, private insurance schemes and employment-specific statutory insurance schemes. Health insurance funds are part of a compulsory social insurance scheme (the sickness funds) for employees with incomes below a certain ceiling. The premium rate is means-tested and fixed. Around 60% of the population is covered in this way. Private insurance schemes cover almost one-third of the population and employment-specific statutory insurance schemes cover around 6% of the population, mainly civil servants, police personnel and the like.
3. *Social Care* is funded from the government budget and covers the entire population. This scheme is for non-serious medical risks and includes family health services and old people's homes.

This system of insurance schemes is in the process of changing, with a move towards a basic insurance package for everyone which will cover at least 85% of the costs of the present health services and related social services. As well as this compulsory basic insurance scheme, which will be means-tested and paid at a fixed premium, there will be a small supplementary insurance which will be optional with a fixed premium.

Patients pay for health care on a fee-for-service basis and are reimbursed by the insurance funds. Health-care fees are based on negotiations between health professionals' representative groups and the government and are tightly controlled by the Central Body for Health Care Charges (*Central Orgaan Tarieven Gezondheidzorg*, COTG).

People who are compulsorily insured are entitled to a number of services including a family doctor, (certain) specialist care, medicines and nursing during the first 365 days of hospitalization. In certain cases, a personal contribution is required. Hospital nursing from the 365th day, nursing homes, homes for the disabled and home nursing are covered by the Exceptional Medical Expenses Compensation Act (AWBZ).

State requirements

The Netherlands is divided into 27 regions for inpatient hospital care. There are norms for the number of beds per 1000 inhabitants for the different categories of hospital service. The number of clinicians per catchment area is also regulated according to medical discipline. All institutions providing health-care services, which are available for those covered by the insurance schemes, must be accredited under the Exceptional Medical Expenses Compensation Act (AWBZ) and must be mentioned in the clause relating to the provision of services in the Health Insurance Act.

For special health facilities licences are required under the Hospital Facilities Act in order to install and to use certain equipment. Facilities listed under this Act include haemodialysis, kidney transplantation, cardiac surgery and neurosurgery, radiotherapy, clinical genetics and genetic counselling, neonatal intensive care and in-vitro fertilization.

Costs for treatment and nursing in psychiatric institutions, nursing homes and institutions for people with learning difficulties are met by AWBZ. Those for treatment and nursing in general and other hospitals are met by the Health Insurance Funds.

Hospital types

Hospitals are designated by the Minister of Health into a number of categories. Such categories include the following:

- university (teaching) hospitals
- general hospitals
- institutions for the deaf or the blind
- nursing homes for the elderly, or physically or mentally ill
- rehabilitation hospitals
- single-specialty hospitals.

Of the non-government run hospitals and services, the majority (over 60%) are not-for-profit and the rest are for profit. Over the past 20 years, the number of nursing homes has increased. Those for the elderly are divided into physical or mental (psycho-geriatric) impairment. There are eight university hospitals, all of which are government rather than private institutions. Around 25 other hospitals are government-run, as are around 20 psychiatric institutions.

Within the different categories, hospitals are further divided into private and public:

- *Private* hospitals are founded by various religious orders and

charitable organizations and function autonomously. Health-care personnel have contracts with the employer.
- *Public* hospitals are established by central, provincial or municipal government and are controlled by central or local government. Health-care personnel are civil servants.

Hospital directors meet regularly on a voluntary basis and work to provide the government with proposals for improving services. Hospitals are run in a competitive market system; technical equipment is sophisticated and medical standards are high.

Access to specialist care

A gatekeeper system applies to socially insured patients but privately insured patients can make an appointment directly with a specialist. Both groups of patients pay almost the same fees.

TRAINING AND TYPES OF POST

Access to medical studies is free but the number of students in the first year of study is limited (*numerus clauses*). Undergraduate training is of 6 years' duration, 4 years pre-clinical and 2 years clinical, during which time the students rotate through the various specialties. The sixth year is spent largely in peripheral hospitals, where students have some responsibility for the daily running of the ward. Dutch medical students (*co-assistenten*) are perhaps more knowledgeable than their British counterparts as far as theory is concerned but the training they receive puts less emphasis on clinical skills.

At the end of the sixth year final examinations are taken and graduates are registered as medical practitioners. They are eligible to begin specialist training without needing to obtain further general experience. Doctors in training have to undergo a probation period which has to be approved by a professionally registered specialist in a teaching hospital. Once the conditions of education and qualification have been fulfilled, the practice of consultants is regulated by registration on a consultants' list.

In the hospital setting, the junior doctor starts out as an *arts-assistant*, with a consultant as supervisor. Admission on to a specialty training programme is on an interview basis and the minimum training period is 5 years. The training programme involves 2 years in a peripheral hospital where the *assistent* gains more general experience, followed by time spent in a teaching hospital. Alternatively, all 5 years may be spent at a teaching hospital. The *assistent* deals with patients on a certain ward rather than having patients scattered throughout the hospital wherever there happens to be a bed. As part of the training requirements, *assistents* are expected to publish at least once and to conduct research at clinical level; the publication of case studies is encouraged. Working hours and on-call duty are shorter than in the UK and so wages are consequently lower. Health-care employees have to pay into the Dutch pension scheme and this money cannot be reimbursed.

Most general practitioners and specialists are self-employed or work as independent practitioners. Consultants in private hospitals are not hospital employees but have a special contract with the hospital, granting them use of outpatient facilities and clinical departments. They are paid on a fee-for-service basis by the patients they treat, rather than receiving a salary. Salaries are paid to doctors in government institutions including teaching hospitals. Hospital consultants form a separate organizational body, with a special set of regulations relating to quality of work, medical ethics and the appointment of new members of staff. They also deal with imposing sanctions in cases of malpractice.

A doctor wishing to become a self-employed specialist must make a 'goodwill' payment in order to enter an established practice. This varies in amount, according to the relevant national association. It is tax-deductible and should be recovered when the practice is sold or the specialist retires. The specialist must also pay for practice administration and assistance — for example, secretaries or technicians. Direct employment contracts with a hospital do not require this 'goodwill' payment.

PRACTICAL POINTS

Euthanasia

This was made legal in the Netherlands in 1992. For assisted death by a medical practitioner to be legally classified as euthanasia rather than murder, the following criteria must be satisfied:

- It must be acknowledged that the patient's suffering is incurable and unbearable.
- The patient's euthanasia request must be well considered and made repeatedly.
- An independent second medical practitioner's opinion must be obtained.
- Euthanasia must be reported to the local coroner.

A national survey conducted in 1996 reported that over half the cases of euthanasia were not being reported. This has led to the development of a support line for GPs which aims to improve the quality of decisions on euthanasia and to optimize the provision of palliative care. The project, known as

Support and Consultation on Euthanasia in the Netherlands (SCEN), has been devised between the Royal Dutch Medical Association (KNMG) and the National General Practitioners' Association (LHV). SCEN will provide a telephone service staffed by trained professionals allowing GPs to discuss the medical and legal aspects of euthanasia and obtain advice.

REGISTRATION

Doctors going to work in the Netherlands must register with the bodies listed in Box 14.3.

BOX 14.3
Organizations involved in Dutch registration

- Inspectie voor de Gezondheidszorg (Dutch Inspectorate for Health Care)
- KNMG (Royal Dutch Medical Association; the equivalent of the BMA)
- Inspector of Health Care in the province where one is to work
- Local mayor
- Local Vreemdelingendienst (foreigner service), which issues residence and work permits.

The Dutch Inspectorate for Health Care is the national competent authority and this body should be contacted for a registration application form and a list of registration requirements. The standard documents required are:

- original diploma
- certificate of nationality (ID certificate or passport)
- certificate of good standing
- certificate of European Equivalency of Training, available from one's native competent authority.

Translations of diplomas from English into Dutch are not required for the Netherlands.

Although no work permits are necessary for EU nationals, applicants from outside the Netherlands have recently been asked for evidence of language proficiency.

FINDING A POST

Posts are advertised in the weekly journal, the *Nederlands Tijdschrift voor Geneeskunde*. Training posts are limited, except in certain fields — for example, paediatrics, anaesthetics and gynecology. It is possible to train for 1 year at medical student level by arranging *co-assistantschap* or a *stage* as part of the Erasmus programme (see p. 30).

LIST OF HOSPITALS

Academisch Ziekenhuis bij de Universiteit van Amsterdam (AZUA)
Academisch Medisch Centrum
Meibergdreef 9
1105 AZ Amsterdam Zuidoost
Tel: 00 31 (0)20 556 9111
Fax: 00 31 (0)20 556 4440
Number of beds: 1050.

Academisch Ziekenhuis Vrije Universiteit (AZVU)
De Boelelaan 1117
1081 HV Postbus 7057
1007 MB Amsterdam
Tel: 00 31 (0)20 444 4444
Fax: 00 31 (0)20 444 4645
Number of beds: 750.

Academisch Ziekenhuis Gronigen
Hanzeplein 1, 9713 GZ
Postbus 30001
9700 RB Groningen
Tel: 00 31 (0)50 361 6161
Fax: 00 31 (0)50 361 4759
Number of beds: 1050.

Academisch Ziekenhuis Leiden
Rijnsburgerweg 10, 2333 AA
Postbus 9600
2300 RC Leiden
Tel: 00 31 (0)71 526 9111
Fax: 00 31 (0)71 522 6478
Number of beds: 870.

Academisch Ziekenhuis Maastricht
P. Debyelaan 25, 6229 HX
Postbus 5800
6202 AZ Maastricht
Tel: 00 31 (0)43 387 6543
Fax: 00 31 (0)43 387 5995 / 7878
Number of beds: 715.

Academisch Ziekenhuis Nijmegen St Radboud
Geert Grooteplein Zuid 10, 6525 GA
Postbus 9101
6500 HB Nijmegen
Tel: 00 31 (0)24 361 1111
Fax: 00 31 (0)24 354 0576
Number of beds: 930.

Academisch Ziekenhuis Rotterdam
Dijkzigt
Dr Molewaterplein 40, 3015 GD
Postbus 2070
3000 CB Rotterdam
Tel: 00 31 (0)10 463 9222
Fax: 00 31 (0)10 463 5306 / 5305
Number of beds: 1260.

Academisch Ziekenhuis Rotterdam
Daniel den Hoed Kliniek
Groene Hilledijk 301
3075 EA Rotterdam
Tel: 00 31 (0)10 439 1911 / 1922
Fax: 00 31 (0)10 486 1058
Number of beds: 150.

Exchange scheme

Academisch Ziekenhuis Utrecht
Interne Geneeskunde
Heidelberglaan 100, 3584 CX
Postbus 85500
3508 GA Utrecht
Tel: 00 31 30 250 9111; 00 31 30 250 73 97
Fax: 00 31 30 254 1474/3064; 00 31 30 251 83 28
Number of beds: 850.

ADDRESSES

Competent authority (*Medical registration*)
Inspectie voor de Gezondheidszorg (Medical Inspector of Health)
Staatstoezicht op de Volksgezondheid
Sir Winston Churchillaan 362
Postbus 5406

2280 HK Rijswijk
Tel: 00 31 (0)70 340 7911

Koninklijke Nederlandsche Maatschappij tot Bevordering der Geneeskunst (KNMG) (*Royal Dutch Medical Association*)
Domus Medica
Lomanlaan 103
3526 XD Utrecht
Tel: 00 31 (0)30 282 3911/81 3713
Fax: 00 31 (0)30 282 3375/26
E-mail: secretar@bureau.knmg
For information about specialist registration and provincial medical registration.

De Geneeskundige Hoofdinspecteur van de Volksgezondheid
(*Medical Inspector of Public Health Care*)
Dr Reijersstraat 10
2265 BM Leidschendam
Sectoral organization all on same premises.

Ordre van Medische Specialisten (*Hospital Specialists' Association*)
Postbus 20057
3502 LB Utrecht
Tel: 00 31 (0)30 282 3300

Rijksinstituut voor Volksgezondheid en Milieu (RIVM) (*Dutch National Institute of Public Health and the Environment*)
Postbus 1
3720 BA Bilthoven

REGISTRABLE QUALIFICATIONS FOR DUTCH DOCTORS GOING ABROAD

The registrable qualification awarded in the Netherlands is the *Universitair getuigschrift van arts* (University certificate of doctors). The country has 14 universities, of which eight have a faculty of medicine. The Free University in Amsterdam is Protestant-Reformist but the other medical schools have no particular religious convictions. The following is a list of licensing bodies (faculties of medicine) and the qualifications granted:

- Universiteit van Amsterdam: *Artsexamen Amsterdam*
- Vrije Universiteit te Amsterdam: *Artsexamen Free U Amsterdam*
- Rijksuniversiteit te Groningen: *Artsexamen Groningen*
- Rijksuniversiteit te Leiden: *Artsexamen Leiden*

- Rijksuniversiteit Limburg te Maastricht: *Artsexamen Maastricht*
- Katholieke Universiteit te Nijmegen: *Artsexamen Nijmegen*
- Rijksuniversiteit te Rotterdam: *Artsexamen Rotterdam*
- Rijksuniversiteit te Utrecht: *Artsexamen Utrecht.*

Further information, particularly for medical students, can be obtained from:

Royal Netherlands Embassy
PCZ (Education)
38 Hyde Park Gate
London SW7 5DP
Tel: 00 44 (0)171 590 3200

An information booklet, entitled 'International Courses in the Netherlands', is available in English.

For longer-term student placements contact:

Foreign Student Service
Oranje Nassaulaan 5
1075 AH Amsterdam
Tel: 00 31 20 6715915,

Send a self-addressed A4 envelope.

For national statistics, check out the OECD website:
http://www.oecd.org/publications/figures/health htmp

Portugal

15

Joined EU: 1986
Area: 92 390 km²
Population (1998): 9.93 million
Population density: 107 persons / km²
Language: Portuguese
Currency: Escudo
Religion: Roman Catholic (97%)
Government: Parliamentary democracy
GDP per head (1994): 11 432 us$
Social security expenditure as % of GDP (1993): 17.3%
Health expenditure as % of GDP (1995): 8.2%
Infant mortality rate (1998): 6.87 deaths per 1000 live births
Average life expectancy at birth (1998): 72.3 (men); 79.3 (women); total 75.7 years
Unemployment (1998): 7%
Doctors per 10 000 population (1995): 29.9
Beds per 10 000 population (1994): 4.1

BACKGROUND

Portugal has undergone considerable development in the last 50 years. The country was under dictatorship rule from the immediate post-war period until 1974 when a democratic government came to power. The present government is right of centre. Parliament is elected every 4 years by proportional representation.

Portugal joined the EU in 1986 and since then has received large amounts of EU aid. In the last decade the economy has been turned around and issues in health and education have also been addressed. Life expectancy has risen, infant mortality has dropped and the emphasis on obstetrics, perinatal and neonatal services continues nationwide. The prevalence of illiteracy is high

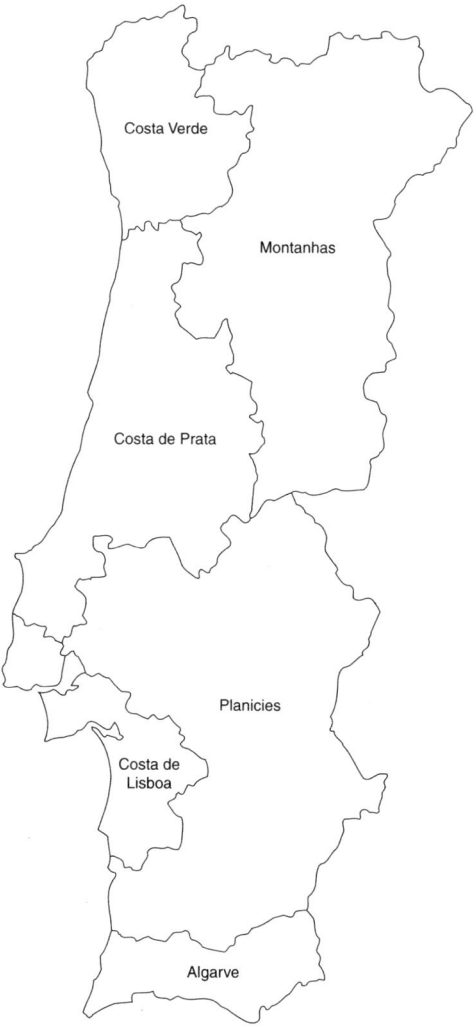

Fig. 15.1 Map of Portugal.

but this is now limited to older members of the community. The EU structural aid programme ends in 1999.

Income tax is self-assessed annually and varies between 15 and 40%. There is also a local tax and VAT. Social security covers old age and disability pensions, cash sickness and maternity benefits, health coverage, unemployment benefits and family allowance.

School education is compulsory for a period of 9 years, from age 5. A decade ago, Portugal had one of the worst literacy rates in Western Europe. It is still lower than that of other EU member states but is now approaching 90%.

LANGUAGE

Portuguese is the national language of Portugal. The letters ã and õ represent the Portuguese nasal vowels. The ç functions as in French, while the combinations lh and nh correspond to Spanish ll and ñ respectively. The letter j is pronounced as in French (not as in Spanish), as is the letter g before e and i. The letter h is always silent.

Galician is a dialect of Portuguese which is spoken by about 3 million people in the northwesternmost part of Spain.

ORGANIZATION OF THE HEALTH SYSTEM

Health care in Portugal was insurance-based until the National Health Service (NHS) reform in 1979. The health system is now government-funded through public taxes and covers all citizens. The population has access to NHS hospitals for emergency treatment and to health clinics for ambulatory care. Public hospital treatment and essential medicines are free. Patients have to pay half the cost of non-essential prescribed medicines and there is a small charge for outpatient treatment by a doctor.

Organization and management are the responsibility of the Ministry of Health. The NHS also covers the autonomous regions of the Azores and Madeira, and in these areas, control of health-care services is the responsibility of the Secretariats for Social Affairs of the regional governments. Around 80% of all health care is provided by the State but other contributions come from charitable bodies and for-profit private clinics.

State health-care services are divided into primary care and specialized treatment. Primary care is provided in local health centres managed by local authorities which are under regional supervision, whereas specialized care requires referral to hospitals. There is no internal competition within the public sector, at health centre or hospital level, although there is discussion as to whether to increase market participation by these services to promote freedom of choice for the consumer.

Private care is not yet fully established in Portugal but certain services are privately run and subsidized by the State. For example, patients seen in the public sector who require laboratory or radiological investigations are often sent to private institutions for these to be performed. The costs are met by the State by way of third-party payment. There is easy access to private sector investigations, with the result that the growth of this field in the NHS has been limited. It is estimated that almost one-third of public health care spending is presently channelled to private providers in this way.

Health care is organized at central, regional and local levels. For health purposes Portugal is divided into 22 regions, each region in turn being divided into municipalities. The government proposes health policies and overlooks service planning and evaluation. The policies are then implemented at regional level by Regional Health Administrations (RHAs).

RHAs are responsible for implementing government policies as well as for integrating national health services with the private sector and for managing contracts with these bodies. They deal with the location and administration of health centres but hospitals have their own executive bodies, so that RHAs play little part in individual hospital management. Health-service professionals are under regional supervision and medical practice, training and research are also dealt with at this level.

Local (municipal) authorities are responsible for primary health care, which is provided in local health centres. Services include preventative medicine and the diagnosis and treatment of disease. The private equivalent is the insurance polyclinic. Portugal spends less than the EC average on health care (GDP is lower; see Fig. 2.1, p. 14), but of this spending, there is a greater proportion directed towards primary health than to hospital care. Due to the development of health centres and primary care in general, the majority of doctors graduating in the last decade have gone into general practice. GPs have to obtain the generalist degree (see 'Training' below) and are contracted to have 1500 patients on their practice lists.

Finance

The health service is funded predominantly from taxation with contributions from users. State hospitals are financed directly by the Ministry of Health according to services provided, whereas private hospitals generally are either funded by religious (non-profit) organizations or are private for-profit institutions. The various hospitals propose budgets and receive allocations of money from the general budget after approval by the Ministry of Health. The amount paid is based on the services provided and is calculated according to basic prices which are fixed annually. In addition to this type of financing, hospitals may have their own sources of income.

Hospital types

The majority of hospitals are public. There is a network of district, central and university-affiliated hospitals, which differ according to size of catchment area and degree of specialization. Patients are referred 'up' the hospital system for increasingly specialized care.

Although hospitals have administrative and financial autonomy, hospital planning is the responsibility of the Ministry of Health and, more specifically, the General Directorate for Hospitals. Within each hospital, there is a board of governors which deals with management. The board consists of a chief executive appointed by the Health Minister, a chairperson, a clinical director and a head of nursing studies.

Access to specialist care

Patients can choose their own GP, although in practice the the options are limited, as GPs do not want to take on more than the 1500 patients they are contracted to care for. Patients have a free choice of hospital but not of specialist. A referral system exists for hospital and specialist care, although in practice patients often present directly to the accident and emergency departments for non-emergency situations in order to bypass the system. There is universal coverage under the NHS but there are flat co-payments for prescriptions and other primary health-care services, as mentioned above.

A small proportion of the public (around 2%) are covered by individual health insurance schemes. Private patients pay the total bill for partial reimbursement later by the NHS. This private sector is likely to expand due to recent tax incentives.

TRAINING AND TYPES OF POST

Access to medical studies is now controlled by way of a *numerus clausus* operating in the first year, in an effort to contain the present problems of unemployment and underemployment. Undergraduate training is of 6 years' duration and an internship period is necessary before a doctor can be fully registered.

There are three official medical careers in Portugal: hospital medicine, general practice and public health. As general practice is considered a specialty, it is necessary to gain the title of 'generalist' (a specialist in general practice). The general practice diploma is awarded after successful completion of a 3-year vocational training programme.

The great majority of doctors are employed by the NHS, where they are salaried employees of the state. Private hospitals are usually staffed by salaried doctors from public hospitals who are paid on a fee-for-service basis when they work privately. A doctor is entitled to engage in private practice if not working full-time in the NHS. Around 50% of NHS employees also practise privately in this way. Very few doctors engage exclusively in private practice, given universal coverage and the quality of health care offered by the NHS.

PRACTICAL POINTS

Medical defence and professional disciplinary procedures

Personal medical indemnity is not compulsory but insurance is available from most insurance companies. The Ordem dos Médicos can provide recommendations on the type of insurance required. The Ordem is responsible for medical disciplinary action but is also available for advice on legal aid for medical professionals.

Private practice

Although there are no restrictions on private practice amongst doctors not working full-time in the NHS, few doctors work exclusively in private practice, as earnings are on a fee-for-service basis and the practice premises must be financed and maintained by the individual doctor. The Ordem dos Médicos has recently established a protocol with the BPA bank (Banco Português do Atlántico) to facilitate raising of the necessary capital. Even so, the demand for private practice by patients is tempered by the universal coverage and the quality of health care available within the NHS.

REGISTRATION

All practising doctors must be members of the Ordem dos Médicos, for which there is an annual membership fee. In order to obtain membership and thus registration, it is necessary to contact the regional branch of the area in which one's employment is to be based. As registration is regional, one needs to have a potential post before applying to the relevant competent authority. The national headquarters of the Ordem dos Médicos in Lisbon (see 'Addresses', below) can supply an application form together with a list of the documents required (notably, proof of nationality, certificate of primary qualification and certificate of registration in one's native EU member state).

FINDING A POST

For doctors wishing to work in the Portuguese NHS there are national rules concerning application and selection. Finding a permanent post is difficult, as vacancies are limited and medical underemployment and unemployment in Portugal are high. NHS vacancies are advertised in the official state journal *Diario da República* and information is also available from the Regional Health Administrations. Posts are given to the best-qualified applicant from amongst those fulfilling the basic legal requirements. It is difficult to organize a post in Portugal independently before arriving in the country but addresses for the above sources of information are available from the Ordem dos Médicos or from the Ministry of Health (see 'Addresses', below).

The *Revista Ordem dos Médicos* and the *Acta Medica Portuguesa* are the main medical journals. They are distributed to all registered doctors by the Ordem dos Médicos.

LIST OF HOSPITALS
Exchange scheme
Faculdade de Medicina de Lisboa
Avenida Prof. Egas Moniz
1600 Lisboa
Tel: 00 351 (0)1 797 4365
Fax: 00 351 (0)1 796 4059

Other hospitals
Hospital de Santa Maria
Avenida Prof. Egas Moniz
1600 Lisboa
Tel: 00 351 (0)1 797 5171
Fax: 00 351 (0)1 790 1219

Faculdade de Medicina do Porto
Rua Prof. Hernani Monteiro
4200 Porto
Tel: 00 351 (0)2 550 3997
Fax: 00 351 (0)2 551 0119

Hospital de São João
Alameda Prof. Hernani Monteiro
4200 Porto
Tel: 00 351 (0)2 527 151 / 527 161
Fax: 00 351 (0)2 525 766

Faculdade de Medicina de Coimbra
Rua Larga
3000 Coimbra
Tel: 0 351 (0)3 928 121
Fax: 00 351 (0)3 923 236

Hospital da Universidade de Coimbra
Avenida Dr Bissaya Barreto
3000 Coimbra

Tel: 00 351 (0)3 940 0400 / 0500 / 0600
Fax: 00 351 (0)3 923 907

ADDRESSES

Competent authority
Ordem dos Médicos (*National Headquarters and Section for Southern Regional Section, Lisbon*)
Avenida Almirante Gago Coutinho 151
1700 Lisboa
Tel: 00 351 (0)1 847 0654
Fax: 00 351 (0)1 847 0467

Ordem dos Médicos (*Central Region*)
Rua D'Alfonso Henriques 39
3000 Coimbra
Tel: 00 351 (0)3 970 1715
Fax: 00 351 (0)3 970 2788

Ordem dos Médicos (*Northern Regional Section*)
Rua Delfim Maia 405
4200 Porto
Tel: 00 351 (0)2 550 7460
Fax: 00 351 (0)2 550 2547

APMCG (*Portuguese Association of General Practitioners*)
(Ministry of Education)
Avenida 5 de Outubro 107
1050 Lisboa
Tel: 00 351 (0)1 795 0330
Fax: 00 351 (0)1 793 3618

REGISTRABLE QUALIFICATIONS FOR PORTUGUESE DOCTORS GOING ABROAD

The registrable qualification granted in Portugal is the *Carta de curso de licenciatura em medicina* (diploma confirming the completion of medical studies), awarded by a university, and the *Diploma comprovativo conclusão do internato geral* (diploma confirming the completion of general internship), awarded by the competent authorities of the Ministry of Health.

There are four universities in Portugal with a faculty of medicine:

- Universidade de Coimbra: *Lic Med Coimbra*
- Universidade de Lisboa : *Lic Med Lisbon*

- Universidade Nova de Lisboa: *Lic Med New U. Lisbon*
- Universidade de Porto: *Lic Med Oporto*.

Further information, particularly for medical students and research workers, is available from:

Departamento do Ensino Superior
Avenida Duque d'Avila 137
1200 Lisboa

Spain

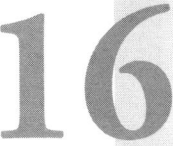

Joined EU: 1986
Area: 504 750 km²
Population (1998) : 39.13 million
Population density: 78 persons / km²
Language: Spanish
Currency: Peseta
Religion: Roman Catholic (99%)
Government: Parliamentary monarchy
GDP per head (1994): 12 654 US$
Social security expenditure as % of GDP (1993): 23.2%
Health expenditure as % of GDP (1995): 7.6%
Infant mortality rate (1998): 6.51 deaths per 1000 live births
Average life expectancy at birth (1994): 73.4 (men); 81.6 (women); total 77.6 years
Unemployment (1997): 21%
Doctors per 10 000 population (1993): 40.8
Beds per 10 000 population (1994): 4.0

BACKGROUND

Although Spain is a popular holiday destination, finding work there can be a challenge for non-Spanish nationals. The pace of life in Spain is typical for the climate and, as with other southern EU countries, administration is a downside. Obtaining registration as a medical practitioner can be a slow-moving and frustrating business and prior knowledge of Spanish is definitely recommended. Another difficulty is unemployment, which is high, and this includes the medical profession. It may be possible to find short-term or locum appointments but more permanent posts are few and far between.

Spain became a constitutional monarchy in 1978 with the end of Franco's authoritarian regime. The King is Head of State. Executive power is vested

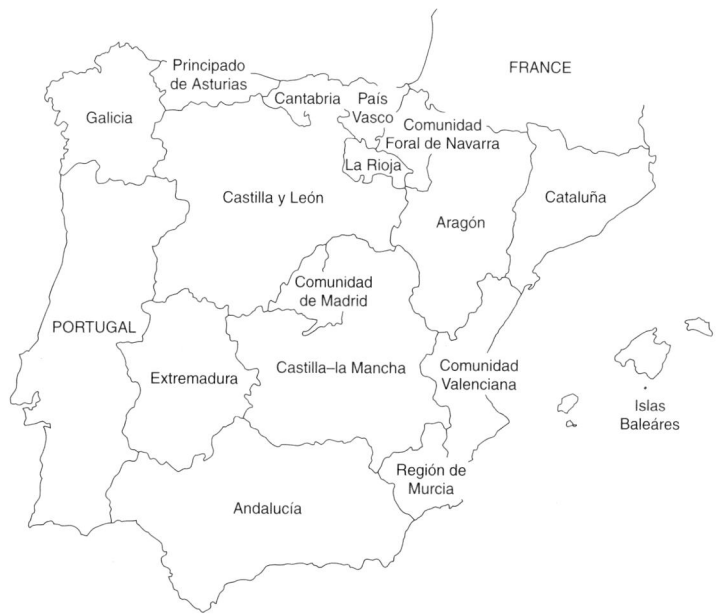

Fig. 16.1 Map of Spain.

in the Prime Minister, who is proposed by the monarch on parliament's approval and is voted into office by the Congress of Deputies. Power is also vested in a Council of Ministers, and the Council of States is a consultative body.

The country is divided into 17 autonomous regions and 50 provinces, which include the Balearic Islands in the Mediterranean and the Canary Islands in the Atlantic. Each of the 17 autonomous regions elects a unicameral legislative assembly. Seven of these regions are composed of only one province; the other ten have two or more. Each province has an appointed governor and an elected council. There are over 8000 municipalities, which are governed by a directly elected council.

Taxation is levied at national and local levels. National taxation includes corporate and personal income tax, VAT, wealth and inheritance and gilt tax. Local taxation includes property and municipal gains taxes as well as various licence fees. Income tax (*Impuesto sobre la Renta de las Personas Físicas, IRPF*) depends on length of time spent in residence in the country, the cut-off being 183 days per year.

Education is free and compulsory from 6–14 years.

LANGUAGE

In addition to Spanish, a number of dialects are spoken in the different regions.

Catalan is a language belonging to the Romance family and is most closely related to Provençal (see 'Language', Chapter 8). It is spoken in north-east Spain and down the coast as far as the province of Valencia. Most of the 7 million speakers of Catalan live in mainland Spain but some 500 000 live in the Balearic Islands, 250 000 in France and 60 000 in Andorra. In provinces where it is spoken, Catalan is co-official with Spanish.

Basque is spoken on both sides of the Spanish–French border by around 1 million people. Of these, around 900 000 are in Spain, in the provinces of Guipúzcoa, Vizcaya and Navarre. Bilbao, the capital of Vizcaya, is the major city of the Basque region. In France, Basque is spoken in the south-western corner, in the department of Pyrénées-Atlantique. Most Basques are bilingual, speaking Spanish or French (or both) in addition to their own language.

In north-west Spain, around 3 million people speak a dialect of Portuguese known as Galician.

ORGANIZATION OF THE HEALTH SYSTEM

Health care in Spain is based on a national health insurance scheme, the *Insalud*. Participation in social insurance is compulsory for all wage-earners and Insalud covers more than 97% of the population for health care within the social security (as opposed to private) sector. Cover includes general and specialist care, medicines and appliances, and ambulances and other transport. Care is free at the point of delivery and co-payments apply only to medicines and only to a sector of the population. Around 40% of the population, mainly the retired, disabled or other vulnerable groups, are exempt from payment. The public sector also includes networks of psychiatric and military hospitals and public health functions such as epidemiology, school health and vaccinations. Dental care is not covered by social security.

A bit of history

Health-care organization has been in the process of reform since the General Health Act of 1986. Prior to the Act, health care was organized into three tiers of service provision comprising primary health-care services, specialist (ambulatory) clinics and hospital services. Admission to hospital for patients was via referral from specialist clinics, except in emergencies. Under this system there was minimal, if any, communication between specialists in ambulatory and hospital sectors.

The General Health Act of 1986 led to the New Care Model. The country's autonomous regions are now divided into Health Areas (*Áreas de Salud*), which are linked to a hospital and provide all the main general and specialist services. Health Areas are further divided into Basic Health Zones (*Zonas Básicas de Salud*), which each have a health centre and deal with primary care. Health-care provision within these geographical boundaries is thus two-tier, with primary care (health centres with primary care teams including GPs and hospital-trained paediatricians) and specialized care. Referral for specialist admission is made by primary care providers (GPs), except in emergencies. Care-providers within a health area must refer patients to the hospital designated for that area. Patients thus have no choice of hospital.

Other features of the Act are listed in Box 16.1.

BOX 16.1
Some features of the Spanish General Health Act 1986

- The Act acknowledged an individual's right to health care. Since 1989, citizens who have evidence that they have no resources are entitled to free health services in the social security sector.
- Public services and institutions were unified into one coordinated system and financing was pooled from the State, the social security system and the autonomous regions.
- The Act also promoted decentralization. Although central government is responsible in the main for laying down general policies and legislation, health-care management and planning is being devolved to autonomous regional level. This has occurred at staggered intervals throughout the country. Some autonomous regions have had this administrative responsibility since the 1980s — Catalonia (1981), Andalusia (1984) and the Basque Region (1988) — while others continue to be directly managed by the Madrid-based Insalud. Health policies devised in this way by the various autonomous regions are coordinated at national level by the Interterritorial Council of the National Health Scheme (Consejo Interterritorial del Sistema Nacional de Salud). The Council is presided over by the Minister of Health and Consumer Affairs.

Private health care

Private health care also exists and runs in parallel with social security services/Insalud. Nationally, around 70% of hospitals are public and 30% are private, but this is variable at regional level. Notably, health sector division in Catalonia is such that 30% of beds are public and 70% are private.

Private care and facilities are available to social security patients under special agreements, as Insalud hospitals do not have all facilities within a given area. Contracting to outside services makes up for around one-fifth of Insalud expenditure.

Hospital types

The Spanish public hospital network which developed in the 1960s and early 1970s, was characterized by large hospitals with around 1000 beds, situated in provincial capitals. Since then, efforts have been made to construct smaller hospitals to provide easier hospital access for the whole population.

Spain's hospitals can be divided into private and public, and of these, public hospitals included in or excluded from Insalud. This has implications for hospital employees, as staff working in the Insalud hospital network are paid a monthly salary for which there is a special statute, similar to civil servants. The majority of employees in other public hospitals outside the Insalud system and those in private hospitals are paid according to each particular hospital's contract of employment and are subject to a general contractual scheme.

Another approach to hospital categorization is by specialty. Hospitals can be single-specialty, general, maternity, psychiatric and care of the elderly or residential. Since the General Health Act, relationships between universities and hospital institutions have been established, with the creation of teaching hospitals and district hospitals linked to a university.

The number of beds per 1000 population is low in Spain by the standards of the majority of European countries, at around 4 beds per 1000 inhabitants. (Of these the majority are in general hospitals, with a lower proportion in specialized and psychiatric hospitals.) This does not include beds for the chronically ill, nursing homes and similar institutions. These services are generally lacking throughout the country. Hospital planning is the responsibility of the autonomous regions, as described above.

Finance

Spanish public hospitals are mainly financed by Insalud, which directly funds the hospitals within its organization, usually based on the number of referrals and length of stay. Funding of hospitals outside the Insalud organization, public and private, comes from sources which include hospital insurance funds, public subsidies, private patients and specific agreements with certain collectives.

Hospital management

Hospitals in regions which have not yet taken over the role of management are run by the Madrid-based Insalud. They operate under the supervision of the Provincial Board of Directors of Insalud.

Access to specialist care

Since the introduction of the New Care Model, Spain has run a gatekeeper system, whereby specialist opinion and hospital admission are arranged by referral from a primary-care provider within the relevant Health Area. For some more specialized services, such as vascular surgery or neurosurgery, patients may have to be seen outside their immediate Health Area and referred to regional or tertiary referral hospitals.

TRAINING AND TYPES OF POST

The doctor:population ratio in Spain is one of the highest in Europe, owing to previous unrestricted admission to the faculties of medicine. A national *numerus clausus* was fixed for those studying medicine in 1979. Since medical studies in Spain last 6 years, the effects of the *numerus clausus* were felt only towards the end of the 1980s. The excess of doctors continues, and at the start of the 1990s it was reckoned that there were around 25 000 unemployed doctors in Spain.

Admission to medical studies is now restricted at entry and is dependent on school grades, together with performance in the national *Selectividad* examination. The 6-year undergraduate course is divided into pre-clinical and clinical phases.

After qualifying, graduates need to sit a national public examination called the *Médico Interne Residente (MIR)* in order to gain a place on a training programme. This includes doctors planning to 'specialize' in general practice in order to obtain the title 'generalist'. The *MIR* is a competitive examination open to any doctor who has trained in an EU member state. Competition is fierce, because of Spain's excess of doctors. Training programmes take around 4–6 years, depending on specialty.

Residence in hospitals for hospital specialists (or in practice for GPs' final year of training) must be recognized by post-graduate training centres. Accreditation for specialty training is dealt with jointly by the Ministry of Health and Consumer Affairs and the Ministry of Education and Science. Once training is complete, a certificate is awarded and the doctor becomes eligible for a specialist post. The medical specialization rate in Spain is high, at around 50%.

Post-graduate examinations are not required for acknowledgement of specialist status but must be taken for appointment to specialist posts. Posts can be categorized according to the duration of employment, as shown in Box 16.2.

> **BOX 16.2**
> **Types of post in Spain**
>
> - *Plazas en propiedad*: permanent posts. Access to these posts involves passing an examination, the *Oposiciones*, which comprises a multiple-choice question paper and an assessment of merit (the *baremo*). The *Oposiciones* are regional rather than national like the MIR and are scored on a points system. Doctors with the highest scores have first choice of the posts available. *Oposiciones* take place at different times depending on region and are held infrequently (sometimes less than once a year in certain regions). *Traslados* are examinations like *oposiciones* but for doctors trying to move from one region to another. For *Traslados*, the number of years of service (*antigüedad*) are taken into account
> - *Interinidades*: posts which become vacant in a certain region between two rounds of *oposiciones*. Doctors in such posts, effectively long-term locums, are called *interinos*
> - *Sustituciones*: shorter-term locum posts

PRACTICAL POINTS

Conditions of work and training programmes

Working hours are generally shorter than in northern European countries owing to the heat. The *siesta* is still practised, although not everywhere. Non-Spanish nationals working in Spain enjoy the work once there but most experience a struggle with the administration to obtain registration. Another problem is recognition of posts or of training between Spain and other countries. For doctors native to the UK, a post in Spain would be considered less beneficial to overall medical training than one in, say, France or the Netherlands. Conversely, the Spanish system does not recognize previous specialty training undertaken elsewhere. It is not possible to work for a few years as a trainee and then expect to 'transfer' to Spain to complete the course. Any doctor fortunate enough to gain a place on a training programme in Spain would have to begin from scratch.

Cardio-pulmonary resuscitation

Spain is a predominantly Catholic country and the attitude to resuscitation status is that patients are *for* resuscitation unless circumstances are exceptional.

Termination of pregnancy

In September 1998, a bill was passed whereby no termination could take place after 12 weeks' gestation except for reasons of maternal physical or mental well-being, rape, incest or fetal malformation.

REGISTRATION

Registration is at regional level. The national competent authority in Madrid can provide a list of regional competent authorities (see 'Addresses', below). The competent authority in the region of future employment must be contacted to obtain a list of the documents required for diploma recognition and a registration application form. Necessary documents vary according to applicant nationality and country of training but in general include:

- primary diploma
- certificate of nationality
- certificate of good standing.

The process of registration can be frustrating but is quicker if all correspondence is carried out in Spanish. Having someone to help on site in Spain is a definite advantage.

If considering establishment in independent practice, it is necessary to contact the local authority (*ayuntamiento*) of the relevant district. This is the case for any business venture. A *gestor administrativo* is an agent available in most towns who can be contracted for a fee to deal with the practice's monetary paperwork on behalf of the practising doctor.

FINDING A POST

Finding a post is difficult, due to the excess of Spanish doctors, but an appointment as locum tenens may be possible to arrange. The regional competent authorities can provide some information about employment availability. Another way of finding short-term employment is to contact the medical personnel staff or head of the relevant department directly in one of the main hospitals in the desired region.

LIST OF HOSPITALS

A full list of hospitals in Spain is available from the following source: *Información Sanitaria y Epidemiología, Catálogo Nacional de Hospitales* (co-publishers: Ministerio de Sanidad y Consumo, Ministerio de la Presidencia, *Boletín Oficial del Estado*). This catalogue gives all hospitals and health clinics for each region in Spain. In each section, the number of hospitals is listed and broken down into public (*públicos civiles*), private (*priv. benéf.* and *priv. no benéf.*) and military (*defensa*) categories. It is available from standard university bookshops in Spain and costs 3600 pesetas but there is also a copy for reference at the Spanish Embassy in London. It is published by:

Imprenta Nacional de Boletín Oficial del Estado
Avenida de Monoteras 54
28050 Madrid

ADDRESSES

Competent authority (*registration at regional level*)
Consejo General de Colegios de Médicos de España
Villanueva 11
28001 Madrid
Tel: 00 34 (0)1 431 7780
Fax: 00 34 (0)1 576 4388

Spanish Embassy
20 Peel Street
London W8 7PD
Tel: 0171 221 0098
Fax: 0171 229 7270
Very helpful. As well as providing hospital details, the embassy publishes an information leaflet on social security for people resident in Spain, with details on unemployment, pensions, health care and taxation. There are also contact addresses to help in the search for non-medical work in Spain from the UK.

Spanish Consulate (*London*)
20 Draycott Place
London SW3 2RZ
Tel: 0171 589 8989
The local Spanish consulate can provide information regarding immigration, residence procedures and the import of household goods and pets for non-Spanish nationals planning to move to Spain.

REGISTRABLE QUALIFICATIONS FOR SPANISH DOCTORS GOING ABROAD

The registrable qualification granted in Spain is the *Título de Licenciado en Medicina y Cirugía* (University degree in medicine and surgery), awarded by the Ministry of Education and Science or the rector of a university. Spain has 27 universities with a faculty of medicine. The following are examples of licensing bodies (faculties of medicine) and the qualifications awarded:

- Universidad de Alcalá de Henares: *LMS Alcalá de Henares*
- Universidad Autónoma de Barcelona: *LMS U Autónoma Barcelona*
- Universidad de Barcelona: *LMS Barcelona*

- Universidad Autónoma de Madrid: *LMS U Autónoma Madrid*
- Universidad Complutense de Madrid: *LMS U Complutense Madrid*.

For further information, the following sources are useful:

Spanish Embassy Education Office
20 Peel Street
London W8 7PD
Tel: 0171 727 2462
Fax: 0171 229 4965
E-mail: conseduca.lon@dial.pipex.com

Instituto Cervantes
102 Eaton Square
London SW1 9AN
Tel: 0171 235 0353
Fax: 0171 235 0329

Sweden

17

Joined EU: 1995
Area: 450 000 km² (39 000 km² of water)
Population (1998): 8.9 million
Population density: 20 persons / km²
Language: Swedish
Currency: Swedish krona
Religion: Evangelical Lutheran (94%)
Government: Constitutional monarchy
GDP per head (1994): 16 230 US$
Health expenditure as % of GDP (1995): 7.2%
Infant mortality rate (1998): 3.93 deaths per 1000 live births
Average life expectancy at birth (1998): 76.5 (men); 82 (women); total 79.2 years
Unemployment (1998): 6.6%
Doctors per 10 000 population (1995): 30.7
Beds per 10 000 population (1994): 6.5

BACKGROUND

Sweden is a constitutional monarchy with a single-chamber parliament (*riksdag*) elected every 4 years. The King is Head of State but has no political power. The country is prosperous and politically stable; the Swedes have not been involved in a war since 1814.

The country is the third largest in the EU and has the second-lowest population density. It is particularly thinly populated in the north, where it is mountainous. The majority of the 8.9 million population live in the south and along the coastal plain. Over four-fifths of Swedes live in urban communities.

Tax is levied at national and local levels and the cost of living is high. Health care is of a high standard. The health system evolved rapidly in the 1990s by way of the Ädel and other health reforms.

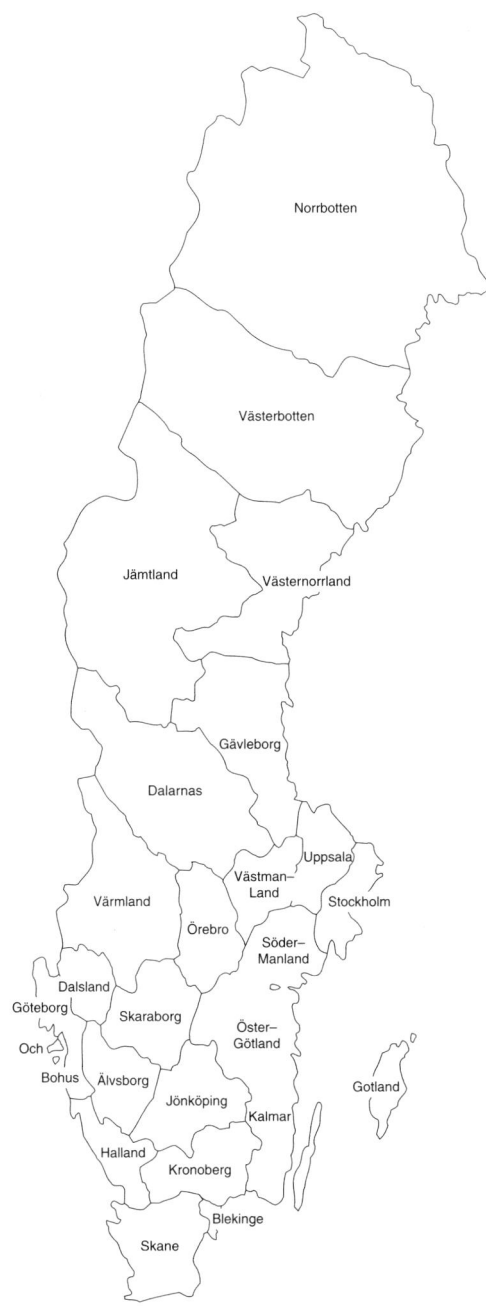

Fig. 17.1 Map of Sweden.

For those driving, imported cars must pass a strict roadworthiness examination, which includes a tough exhaust emission test. After 2 years of residence, a Swedish driving licence must be obtained.

School education is compulsory for a period of 9 years, starting from age 6 or 7 years.

LANGUAGE

Swedish is the most widely spoken of the Scandinavian languages. In addition to the 8.9 million Swedish nationals, there are around 300 000 speakers on the south-western and southern coasts of Finland. The alphabet consists of the 26 letters of the English language plus å, ä and ö. The ä and ö distinguish Swedish from Norwegian and Danish, which use æ and ø respectively for these sounds.

ORGANIZATION OF THE HEALTH SYSTEM

A bit of history

In the last 30 years, the Swedish health service has undergone a series of radical changes. In the 1960s there were marked inequalities in health-care provision between high and low socio-economic groups. As this was felt to be based on the cost of care and treatment, consultation fees were reduced and the imbalance became less marked in the 1970s and 1980s. In the early 1990s, however, discrepancies began to reappear and further reforms were introduced.

In 1991, the 'freedom of choice' policy was adopted by the Swedish Federation of County Councils. This entitled patients to choose their own primary-care centre and permitted, in addition, direct access (that is, without GP referral) to all acute hospital care within a patient's particular county.

In 1992, the year of the Ädel reforms, responsibility for community care of the elderly and other non-acute services was transferred from county council (regional) to municipal (local) level. The goal was to relieve blocking of acute beds, and community-care providers were fined for not being able to accept patients back from acute hospitals. This reduced the percentage of GDP spent on health care and consequently stabilized the health-care budget.

In 1995, the right of establishment of private specialists was withdrawn by the government. Those already in practice could continue but no more establishments were allowed. In 1996 there were further reforms in health-service organization, with moves towards cooperation and purchasing, similar to those which had occurred in the British NHS some years before. These market-style reforms included purchaser–provider splits and performance-related payment systems and were implemented at county level.

The Swedish health system is now characterized by decentralization, with national policies being implemented by government and administered at regional and local level. The government deals with national financial control, legislation and the granting of permits and sanctions. The majority of research and training is also under government control, although they are increasingly being managed at council level. Regional (county council) and local (municipal) authorities are self-governing groups and the system is notable in that it is not hierarchical.

County councils are responsible for Sweden's health care in both primary-care and specialist settings. The councils are funded by local income tax levied by the councils themselves and paid by residents. There are 23 county councils and 3 large municipalities, each with populations of between 60 000 and 1.7 million. Each county council is governed by a local council which is elected every 4 years, concurrent with government elections. The Federation of County Councils (*Landstingsförbundet*) was formed by the county councils to represent them in negotiations with national government on political and economic issues and with respect to trade unions.

Municipalities are responsible for social services, care of the elderly and disabled, psychiatric services and schools. There are 288 municipalities, each dealing with populations of between 5000 and 70 000. They are governed by locally elected councils. The municipalities have formed the Swedish Association of Local Authorities to represent them on a national level.

The Federation of County Councils and the Swedish Association of Local Authorities are not subordinate to the government nor to the central administrative agencies, although they work according to national guidelines (see Fig. 17.2).

Before the Ådel reforms, responsibility for the long-term care of elderly and disabled persons was shared between the municipalities and the county councils. Now that the municipalities are entirely responsible for this type of care, the county councils must be reimbursed by municipal authorities for the cost of continued short-term geriatric care of patients whose medical treatment has been completed. Since 1995, this also applies to psychiatric patients.

At national level, the Swedish ministries are relatively small compared to those in other EU countries. The Ministry of Health and Social Affairs (*Socialdepartementet*) deals with the social insurance system, social security, health and medical care, drug and alcohol abuse and services for special-need groups. The different programmes are implemented by a number of central administrative agencies (see Box 17.1). The National Institute of Public Health (*Folkhälsoinstitutet*), one such agency, was established in 1992 and is

SWEDEN

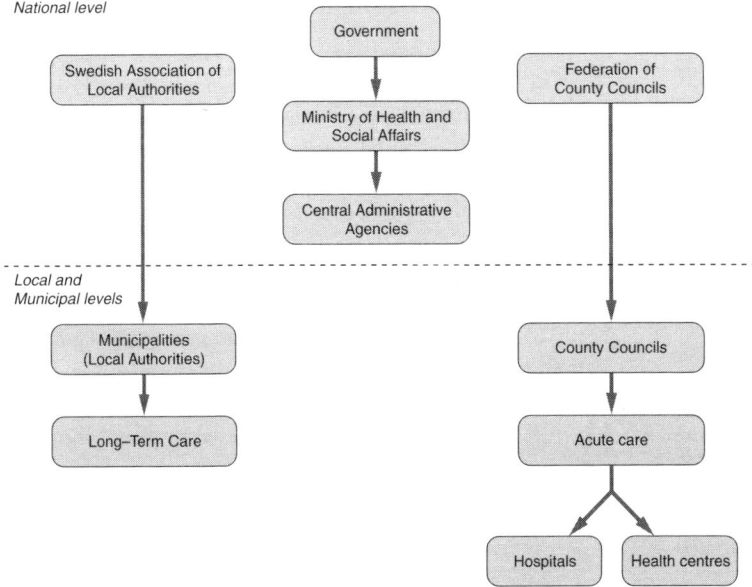

Fig. 17.2 Structure of the Swedish health-care system.

BOX 17.1
Government administrative agencies in Sweden

- National Board of Health and Welfare (Socialstyrelsen)
- National Medical Disciplinary Board (Hälso-och sjukvårdens ansvarsnämnd)
- National Social Insurance Board (Riksförsäkringsverket)
- National Institute of Public Health (Folkhälsoinstitutet)
- Medical Products Agency (Läkemedelsverket)

---

responsible for local health promotion and disease prevention at national level. The National Board of Health and Welfare (*Socialstyrelsen*), another administrative agency, supervises and monitors the public health activities of the county councils and municipalities. The National Epidemiology Centre is part of the Socialstyrelsen and is responsible for managing the national register of diseases and cause of death. Other functions of the board include monitoring health and medical care services and dealing with patient injury reports, as described later in this chapter.

Finance

Around 75% of funding comes from tax levied by county councils, considered as universal public health insurance covering medical care costs for individuals; 12% comes from grants from national government; 3% from patients' fees; and 10% from interests and other income (see Fig. 17.3).

Hospital types

Hospitals can be classified into regional, central county and district county according to size and degree of specialization. Around 95% of short-term beds are provided by the county councils. The number of private hospitals increased in the 1990s but there are few private hospitals for short-term care. They are relatively small compared to county council establishments and so make up a very small percentage of total hospital beds. With the Ådel reforms, the number of hospital beds in Sweden was able to be reduced, as non-acute treatment was transferred to community-based care.

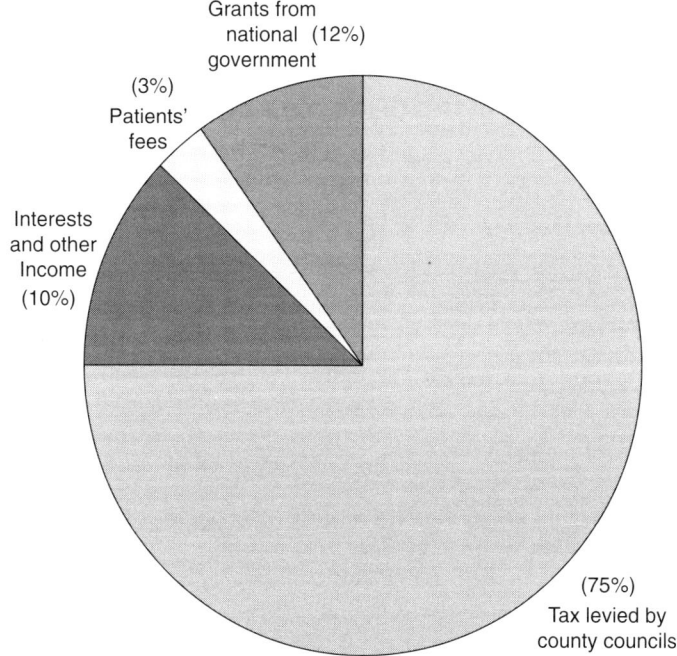

Fig. 17.3 Breakdown of Swedish health-care finance shown as a pie chart. The tax levied by county councils, making up the majority of health care finance is considered as universal public health insurance for individuals' medical care cost.

Duties of each hospital type are divided as follows:

- Regional hospitals provide the most highly specialized care. They are administered by county councils, which operate in six medical care regions. Each region serves a population averaging over 1 million. There are nine such regional hospitals in Sweden. They also function as research and teaching hospitals and are affiliated to medical schools. Each regional hospital has around 900 short-term beds.
- Central county hospitals are the next level down. There is one central county hospital per county council area. Between 15 and 20 specialties are provided and each hospital has an average of 450 beds.
- District county hospitals provide at least four services, including medicine, surgery, radiology and anaesthetics, and have an average of around 130 beds.

Health care and treatment in hospital is provided without patient charges, as taxes levied by the county councils are considered as universal public health insurance. For ambulatory (out-patient) care, a charge is made per visit. Set limits for doctors' fees are established by national government and vary between county councils. Treatment for children under school age and antenatal checks are without charge. There are co-payments for prescribed drugs in ambulatory but not inpatient care.

Primary care which is provided in health centres in Sweden is organized into primary care districts, each with one or more local health centres. There are around 950 such districts in the country. GPs who work in these health centres must possess the qualification of 'specialist in family medicine'. Patients have the right to choose their own GPs and hospitals.

Most physicians (GPs and specialists) are salaried, whether they work in primary care centres or hospitals. The proportion of GPs is low in relation to the total number of doctors at around 20% but there are still plenty to go around, given the total number of doctors in relation to population. Around 90% of all physicians are employed in the county council sector. The establishment of private practice under the social security system is possible only with the consent of the county council concerned. Private health care is limited, with fewer than 10% of all physicians working full-time in private practices. For dental care, over half is carried out privately.

Access to specialist care

There is no gatekeeper system, although referral may be required if patients wish treatment outside their own county council.

TRAINING AND TYPES OF POST

Medical education is financed entirely by the State. Admission to medical school requires graduation from secondary school with subjects in natural science. Basic medical training is for a period of 5½ years, with at least 40 weeks of full-time studies per year. The course is divided into pre-clinical, preparatory and clinical stages. After graduation from medical school, there is a compulsory training programme (internship) of 21 months in order to become a registered doctor. This includes 6 months' surgery, 6 months' internal medicine, 3 months' psychiatry and 6 months' family medicine. After successful completion of the programme, which involves written and practical examinations, the doctor obtains full registration from the National Board of Health and Welfare, and is then entitled to apply for a specialist training post.

Specialist training lasts for a minimum of 5 years, depending on specialty. Assessment of the trainee is the responsibility of the head of department in the relevant specialty. Once training objectives have been achieved, the head of department issues an official certificate. The doctor must then apply to the National Board of Health and Welfare for formal qualification as a specialist to be granted.

Sweden complies with EU recommendations to allow post-graduate medical training in a member state other than that of undergraduate studies. Programmes are open to qualified doctors who require a pre-registration service before obtaining one of the listed recognized qualifications. They are broadly divided into the internship programmes of 21 months' duration and short-term medical appointments (locum tenens) in a subordinate position. Applicants must pass a language test following a formal decision of the National Board of Health and Welfare, however, before they are eligible for such appointments.

PRACTICAL POINTS

Terms and conditions

Working hours are generally 40 per week. Out-of-hours duty is paid and nights or weekends on call are compensated with payment or time off, depending on the number of hours in the basic working week. Salaries and general terms and conditions of employment are negotiated between the Federation of County Councils and the Swedish Medical Association (SMA), although terms can be further negotiated at local level (individual county councils and the local branch of the SMA). Between 90 and 95% of Swedish doctors are members of the SMA. The Association is useful for bargaining with respect to conditions of employment but is also active in education and international relations.

Medical defence and professional disciplinary procedures

The National Board of Health and Welfare is responsible for monitoring health and medical care services at county council, local authority or private level, including injury or disease in connection with medical care or treatment. Reports of patient injury received by the Board are referred to the National Medical Disciplinary Board (*Hälso-och sjukvårdens ansvarsnämnd*). This government agency may impose disciplinary sanctions or even remove the doctor in question from the medical register.

All patients (public and private) are covered by a special 'patient insurance' paid by the county councils and other care-providers, which operates on a no-fault principle. The insurance provides economic compensation for injury in connection with medical treatment or care, without having to prove that the injury was the result of negligence. The requirement is that the relation of cause and effect between treatment and damage be established, and that the damage sustained is not a 'normal' risk of the medical procedure in question. The doctor responsible for the treatment is obliged to inform the patient if he or she considers that damage has occurred, and also to assist the patient in applying for compensation.

Doctors are still, however, recommended to have complementary private liability insurance. The premiums are low, as the 'patient insurance' covers almost all cases of demands for compensation.

Drugs

The National Corporation of Swedish Pharmacies (*Apoteksbolaget*) is owned by the national government. The Corporation possesses the sole and exclusive right to retail drugs to the general public and to hospitals. Drugs listed in a specially compiled formulary are refunded by national health insurance when used in treatment but not for prevention. The Medical Products Agency (*Läkemedelsverket*) is responsible for regulating drugs and other pharmaceutical products and for providing drug information.

REGISTRATION

The National Board of Health and Welfare is the Swedish competent authority. To register, one needs to request an application form and submit a completed version, together with the following documents:

- evidence of primary qualification
- certificate of good standing with the competent authority of the native member state (not required for doctors coming from another EU member state)
- curriculum vitae.

On registration, a licence to practise medicine is issued, together with information emphasizing that a knowledge of the Swedish language and *of all relevant medical legislation is required*. The National Board of Health and Welfare also provides details of suitable language courses, which is useful as future employers (including the county councils) are entitled to demand proof of linguistic and legal competence before awarding a post as a medical practitioner.

Sweden does not maintain the nationality requirement of EEC Directive 93/16/EEC but this policy has no legal consequence in relation to other member states.

FINDING A POST

Vacant posts are advertised in the Swedish medical journal (*Läkartidningen*) and official publications. At university hospitals, contracts for periods of 6 years are common, but shorter appointments are available as locum tenens.

In the last 25 years, the number of Swedish physicians has almost trebled and at present there is a surplus. In addition, expansion of the health sector has ceased and there is strong competition for training posts, particularly for specialist training.

LIST OF HOSPITALS

Södersjukhuset
11883 Stockholm
Tel: 00 46 (0)8 616 1000

Sahlgrenska Universitetssjukhus
41345 Göteborg
Tel: 00 46 (0)31 773 1000

Norrlands Universitetssjukhus
1 Umeå
90185 Umeå
Tel: 00 46 (0)90 785 0000

Universitetssjukhuset
1 Lund
22185 Lund
Tel: 00 46 (0)4 617 1000

Universitetssjukhuset
1 Linköping
58185 Linköping
Tel: 00 46 (0)1 322 2000

SWEDEN

Akademiska Sjukhuset
1 Uppsala
75185 Uppsala
Tel: 00 46 (0)1 866 3000

List of faculties of medicine (Medicinska Faculteten)

Karolinska Institutet
Box 60400
S-104 01 Stockholm
Tel: 00 46 (0)8 728 64 00
Fax: 00 46 (0)8 31 03 43

Uppsala Universitet
Box 256 S-751 05 Uppsala
Tel: 00 46 (0)18 18 25 00
Fax: 00 46 (0)18 18 18 58

Universitetet i Linköping
S-581 83 Linköping
Tel: 00 46 (0)13 22 20 00
Fax: 00 46 (0)13 10 44 95

Lunds Universitet
Box 1703
S-221 01 Lund
Tel: 00 46 (0)46 222 00 00
Fax: 00 46 (0)46 222 45 40

Göteborgs Universitet
Box 33050
S-400 33 Göteborg
Tel: 00 46 (0)31 773 10 00
Fax: 00 46 (0)31 82 58 92

Umeå Universitet
S-901 87 Umeå
Tel: 00 46 (0)90 16 50 00
Fax: 00 46 (0)90 16 76 60

ADDRESSES

Competent authority (*National Board of Health and Welfare*)
Socialstyrelsen

S-106 30 Stockholm
Tel: 00 46 (0)8 783 30 00
Fax: 00 46 (0)8 783 34 20

Swedish Medical Association
Sveriges läkarförbund
Box 5610
S-114 86 Stockholm
Tel: 00 46 (0)8 790 33 00
Fax: 00 46 (0)8 10 31 44; 00 46 (0)8 20 47 18

Läkartidningen (*Swedish Medical Journal*)
Box 5603
S-114 86 Stockholm
Tel: 00 46 (0)8 790 33 00
Fax: 00 46 (0)8 20 76 19

Swedish Society of Medicine
Svenska Läkaresällskapet
Box 738
S-101 35 Stockholm
Tel: 00 46 (0)8 440 88 60
Fax: 00 46 (0)8 440 88 99

Federation of Swedish County Councils
Landstingsförbundet
Box 70491
S-107 26 Stockholm
Tel: 00 46 (0)8 702 43 00
Fax: 00 46 (0)8 702 45 90

REGISTRABLE QUALIFICATION FOR SWEDISH DOCTORS GOING ABROAD

The registrable qualification granted in Sweden is the *Läkarexamen* (university diploma in medicine), awarded by a university faculty of medicine, and a *Certificate of practical training*, issued by the National Board of Health and Welfare.

Sweden has six universities, all of which have a faculty of medicine. The following is a list of these and the qualifications awarded:

- Universitetit i Göteborg: *Läkarexamen Göteborg*
- Universitetit Linköping: *Läkarexamen Linköping*
- Universitetit Lund: *Läkarexamen Lund*

- Karolinska Institutet, Stockholm: *Läkarexamen Stockholm*
- Universitetit Umeå: *Läkarexamen Umeå*
- Universitetit Uppsala: *Läkarexamen Uppsala*.

For further information, the Swedish Institute is a good source:

Svenska Institutet
Box 7434
S-103 91 Stockholm
Tel: 00 46 8 789 20 00
Fax: 00 46 8 20 72 48
E-mail: si@si.se
(Website): http://www.si.se

United Kingdom 18

Joined EU: 1973
Area: 244 820 km^2
Population (1995): 58.3 million (England 48.7; Wales 2.9; Scotland 5.1; N. Ireland 1.6)
Population density: 238 persons / km^2
Language: English
Currency: Pound sterling
Religion: Anglican (46%); Roman Catholic (15%)
Government: Constitutional monarchy
GDP per head (1994): 16 442 US$
Social security expenditure as % of GDP (1993): 26.7%
Health expenditure as % of GDP (1995): 6.9%
Infant mortality rate (1998): 5.87 deaths per 1000 live births
Average life expectancy at birth (1994): 74.6 (men); 80 (women); total 77.2 years
Unemployment (1997): 5.5%
Doctors per 10 000 population (1994): 15.6
Beds per 10 000 population (1994): 4.9

BACKGROUND

The United Kingdom comprising Great Britain, (England, Scotland and Wales) and Northern Ireland is a popular destination for overseas doctors, from EU countries and beyond, as English is a common second language and the standard of medicine is considered to be high. Having some grasp of English is mandatory amongst all health professionals, as the majority of medical and scientific literature is in English, even if the articles are printed abroad.

It may come as a surprise to British junior doctors but, compared to some of their continental European counterparts, they have a pretty good deal. Over the past 10 years in Britain, concerted efforts have been made to protect

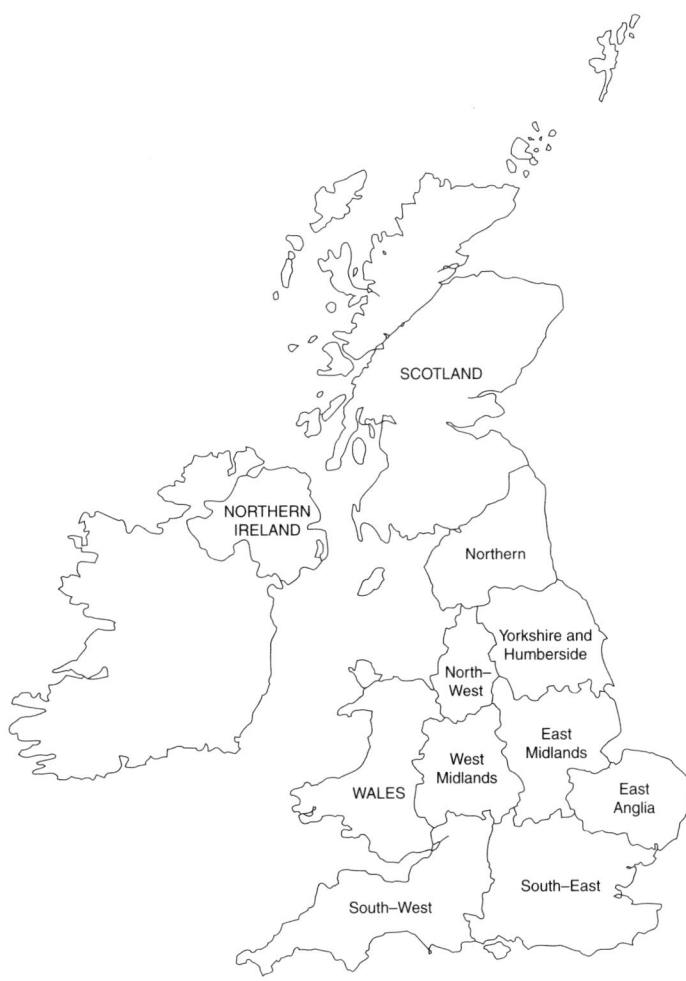

Fig. 18.1 Map of the United Kingdom including the regional divisions of England.

doctors in training from being 'abused', with a particular focus on the number of hours worked per week and the duties performed. Out-of-hours duty is now paid according to the amount of sleep expected, from 'Class 1' to 'Class 3' *Additional Duty Hours* (ADHs), and certain tasks — for example, administration of intravenous drugs — are now generally performed by nursing staff. In some posts, shift-working rotas have been introduced as a measure to keep the working week under 70 hours.

British teaching methods have a strong emphasis on clinical skills and this is held in high regard by doctors trained elsewhere. Bedside teaching of students is a requirement of all junior doctors based at teaching hospitals and students are also taught in small tutorial settings. As imaging techniques are not always easily available, particularly in the district general setting (see below), clinical skills are important.

Despite a reputation for xenophobia, Britain is becoming more accommodating to doctors from overseas. The pie chart (see Fig. 18.2) shows the percentage of doctors from other EU states who are granted full registration with the national competent authority, the General Medical Council. Just under 10% of the total population is made up of ethnic minorities and, as well as EU nationals, visa-free entry to Britain is available to citizens of eastern European states and what is now the Hong Kong Special Administrative Region of China. The larger towns and cities are increasingly cosmopolitan and if the notorious British cuisine becomes too much, there should be adequate continental European or other alternatives.

The United Kingdom is currently in the process of constitutional reform. Grudges have been held intermittently between the Scots and the English since political union in 1707. One concern for the former was that they felt their views were under-represented in a parliament based in the south of England in Westminster, London. In a referendum held in September 1997, the people of Scotland voted 'yes' to reinstating a Scottish parliament and members were elected to this and to a new Welsh assembly in Cardiff in May 1999.

Here is not the place to promote national spirit nor to speculate on future developments but doctors should note the fact that the Scottish parliament in Edinburgh will take decisions on health spending, likely to take up a third of the overall Scottish budget. Of relevance to EU citizens, it is possible one day that Scotland and Wales will consider applying for individual EU membership.

At present, though, it is early days.

Politics aside (well, in theory), the island's demography is closely linked to its geography. In each of England, Scotland and Wales, the northern regions are more hilly than those in the south and the population in these regions is consequently smaller and more rural-based. The majority of commercial centres are located in the southern regions of each country, although in the north of England several large towns exist as centres of industry. Transport services between towns and villages are generally of high standard.

LANGUAGE

English is the official language of the United Kingdom. Others include the Celtic languages of Welsh and Gaelic. Although the former is spoken by less than 25% of the Welsh population (around 600 000 people), in some areas

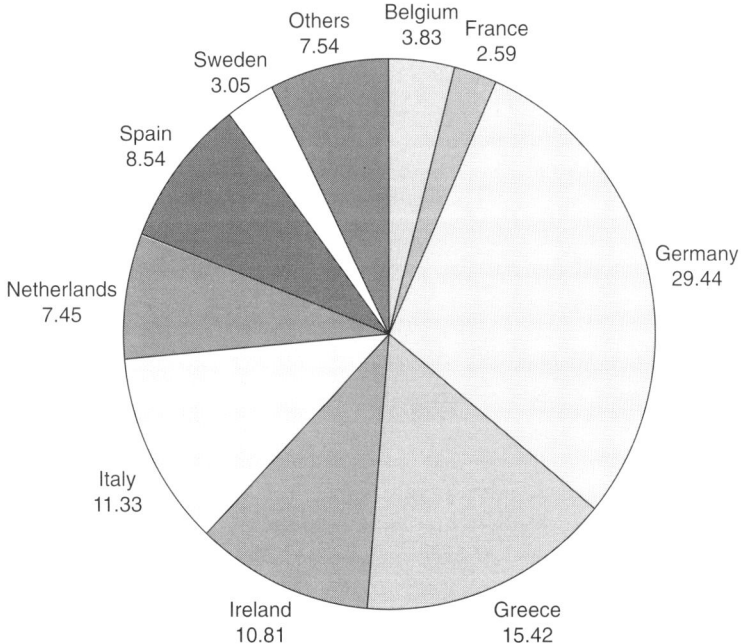

Fig. 18.2 Pie chart showing GMC registration awarded to EEA nationals (1997).

of Wales it is considered to be the first language. Having Welsh is therefore an advantage for work in Wales but the BMA's Welsh Council has made it policy that criteria for awarding posts are based on potential employees' medical competence rather than on language skills. Scottish Gaelic is spoken by only 75 000 people or around 1.5% of the population of Scotland and has no official status. Irish Gaelic is mentioned in Chapter 11.

ORGANIZATION OF THE HEALTH SYSTEM

The UK's National Health Service (NHS) was set up in 1948 as a means of providing comprehensive health care to all, free at the point of delivery. Since its inception, the health service has undergone extensive changes, particularly in the 1990s, and plans for further restructuring are currently under way. Scotland and Northern Ireland have historically had different but comparable systems to England and Wales. Some of the recent restructuring has led to a more unified system between the countries but this again is likely to change with the introduction of national parliaments. The following is a brief description of how the current health-care system is structured and how it is likely to change.

A bit of history

Responsibility for the NHS shifted in 1988 from the Department of Health and Social Security to the Department of Health. The Department sets general policy guidelines and, through the Health Secretary, is accountable for the NHS to parliament. Although the Department is in charge of NHS funding, matters such as professional discipline and training are the responsibility of the national competent authority, the General Medical Council (GMC).

Below central or government level, health care is dealt with at regional and local levels. England is divided into regional health authorities and Wales is a region in its own right. Each Regional Health Authority (RHA) has a board which comprises executive and non-executive members, headed by a non-executive chairperson who is appointed by the Secretary of State. Health service resources, allocated by the Department of Health, are distributed by the RHAs to District Health Authorities (DHAs) and Family Health Service Authorities (FHSAs). Each DHA has a population of between 250 000 and 300 000. FHSAs have similar boundaries but may be larger. The FHSAs are responsible for the management of out-of-hospital services provided by general practitioners, general dental practitioners, pharmacists and opticians. Resource allocation between authorities is carried out according to regionally and nationally determined policies and the RHAs are in charge of monitoring the performance of these authorities at district level. The RHAs are responsible to the Secretary of State, thereby providing a link between government and district level.

In April 1991, fundamental changes in health-care organization took place, altering the role of RHAs. With the introduction of the NHS and Community Care Act, *provision* was separated from *purchase* of health care (including hospitals, community nursing, etc.) and an internal market was introduced in which providers compete for contracts. When the Act was introduced, the RHAs had a key role in overseeing the change from the old hierarchical system to a market system of management, and in developing the contracting process within this market system. This involved setting standards, ensuring effective use of resources and developing a framework for health-service purchasers.

The role of DHAs also changed with the Act in that they became responsible for purchasing (also known as *commissioning*) health services on behalf of their resident populations. The DHAs work jointly with FHSAs to assess the needs and preferences of their population. They then place contracts with providers of health services, in order to meet those needs according to national and regional guidelines. They are also responsible for promoting good health in their resident populations and for monitoring providers' performance against contracts in terms of quality of service and value for money.

These structural changes also led to the development of NHS Trusts. These are hospitals or other health service units which have opted out of DHA and RHA control and have become accountable directly to the Department of Health. Contracts for the provision of health services may thus be placed by the DHAs with directly managed units, NHS Trusts or with private sector hospitals, introducing an element of competition among health-service providers and thereby encouraging the provision of high standards. (See also GP fundholding, p. 202.)

In Scotland, the RHA equivalent is the Regional Health Board. These boards are responsible for hospital and family practitioner services and are accountable to the Scottish Office for the provision of these. Local management units are directly accountable to the Regional Boards with no intermediate district level. Social Services Boards are the equivalent in Northern Ireland.

Future developments

The current system of health-care provision is likely to change in the next few years. Each country within the UK is to have its own parliament and this may lead to the devolution of health-care policy. The new Scottish Parliament, for example, after its first 'shadow' year, will have the power to influence spending on health care, to change doctors' training and education, and to decide on terms and conditions for health professionals working in the NHS. The new Parliament will not, however, be able to regulate the medical profession (the role of the GMC), decide on the control of medicines, or pass legislation on ethical issues. Professional networks will continue to be UK-wide, and will monitor standards of practice and training and how staff are treated.

Finance

The majority (80%) of NHS funding comes from general taxation. Other sources include co-payments, mainly for pharmaceutical products and appliances and dental services, and National Insurance. In 1994, NHS expenditure accounted for 15% of total public expenditure, totalling £40 billion. Of this, over two-thirds was allocated to hospital and community health services. The remainder went towards primary care and other services — for example, ambulance services. (Figures vary depending on the definition of primary health care.) Pharmaceutical products account for around 10% of total NHS gross expenditure. A charge is levied for prescribed drugs but exemption procedures exist for certain groups such as the elderly, those with chronic diseases or those on low incomes, so that some 80% of prescribed medication is issued without charge.

Before the NHS and Community Care Act, allocations to health-care providers were based on the historic cost of service delivery. Since the Act, money available to the NHS has been allocated according to the number of residents in each DHA, with adjustments to compensate for large populations of people at extremes of age or the socially deprived. With the market system, money flows with the patient so that, for example, payment for a certain patient's specialist care in a regional centre will come from that patient's resident DHA, even if the referral centre is outside the authority's catchment area.

Hospital types

A variety of hospitals exist, and may be categorized according to their size, degree of specialization, and whether or not they are linked to a university. There are more than 30 teaching hospitals within the UK which provide pre-qualification training for doctors and have research facilities. There are also regional single-specialty centres but these tend to be for post-graduate training.

Hospital beds are provided for continuing care services (elderly and psychiatric), but the increasing emphasis on community care has meant that the majority of hospital services lie within the acute sector. The size of acute hospitals is variable, from small community to 1000-bed teaching hospitals.

The concept of district general hospitals (DGHs) was introduced in the 1960s. These hospitals provide a basic range of services to the local catchment area and 'refer up' to regional centres for more specialist (tertiary) care. The link between DGHs and teaching hospital centres is also valuable for training purposes, as district hospitals provide more general experience for medical students and junior doctors.

There is no formal accreditation process for acute hospital services. There is, however, a need for the accreditation of post-graduate training posts and this encourages the maintenance of standards in each hospital. If the approval of posts is withdrawn, the number of junior medical staff applications will fall.

Medical audit has been introduced since the NHS and Community Care Act and the development of the contracting process in an effort to maintain and improve service quality.

Hospital management

NHS Trusts, which have opted out of DHA and RHA control, report directly to the Department of Health. They can create their own management structures and employ staff on their own terms and conditions. They are self-governing and run by a board of executive and non-executive directors.

Access to specialist care

The UK operates a gatekeeper system. Patients can choose their own general practitioner (GP) and everyone in the UK should be registered with one. Most GPs now work in group practices rather than individually, so that 24-hour cover can be provided between partners. Patients do not have access to acute NHS services without a GP's referral, unless they are well known to a specialist service — for example, patients with certain chronic diseases.

The development of NHS Trusts also saw the arrival of GP fundholders. These are GPs who are given an allocation of funds to buy hospital services on behalf of their patients, stimulating competition amongst providers (as described above) but also promoting the integration of primary and secondary care. GPs are eligible to opt out if they have more than 5000 patients (3000 for community services fundholding) on their practice lists. A defined range of services can be purchased, including outpatient services, diagnostic tests and certain inpatient and day-case treatments, mostly elective surgery. From April 1999, however, the purchase of NHS services became the responsibility of Primary Care Groups rather than GP fundholders. Primary Care boards are made up of GPs, nurses, and social services and community representatives.

TRAINING AND TYPES OF POST

Access to medical studies is limited from day one. There are around five applicants for each university place and each place is awarded depending on examination results ('A' levels or Scottish Highers) on leaving school and on performance at interview.

Undergraduate training is for a period of 5 or 6 years, depending on medical school and on whether or not the student takes an intercalated degree. After graduation, the primary qualification is awarded and provisional registration is granted by the GMC. The title 'doctor' can be used but a period of 12 months (6 months in surgery, 6 months in medicine) must be spent working as a pre-registration house officer (PRHO) before full registration can be obtained. These posts are salaried and the PRHO is licensed to prescribe medication.

After the PRHO year, the doctor automatically becomes a senior house officer (SHO) in a chosen specialty (medicine, surgery, obstetrics and gynaecology, anaesthetics, etc.). For further medical and surgical specialization, Membership of one of the Royal Colleges must be obtained (see Box 18.1). The doctor thus remains at SHO level for between 2 and 3 years.

Once Membership of a college is obtained and a post becomes available, specialization can begin as specialist registrar (SpR). (SpR posts are currently

> **BOX 18.1**
> **Membership of the Royal Colleges (UK and Ireland)**
>
> Membership of one of the Royal Colleges is required in the UK and Ireland before a specialist training post can be awarded. Membership is obtained by passing the examination of the relevant college, which is in two or three parts depending on discipline. Eligibility to sit each part depends on the time spent in practice post-qualification and on the procedures carried out. Pass rates for these examinations are not available from the Royal Colleges but word has it they are in the order of 30%. They are expensive to sit and demoralizing to fail but unfortunately unavoidable if one is planning a specialist career.
>
> For MRCP (Membership of the Royal College of Physicians), the examination is in two parts:
>
> - Part I is a multiple-choice question paper which is negatively marked (that is, a wrong answer results in a point being deducted rather than simply not being awarded). It takes place three times a year and costs £200 to sit.
> - Part II can be taken once Part I has been obtained, provided the doctor has been in hospital practice for a minimum of 18 months with full GMC (competent authority) registration. There are written and clinical sections. The written section of Part II comprises short-answer questions, questions based on photographs, and 'grey cases'. Grey case questions describe a patient's symptoms and investigation results without offering a diagnosis and ask questions about further management. The written paper costs £200 and successful candidates are then invited to sit the clinical section. The clinical examination is divided into a long case, with 1 hour spent taking a history, examining a patient and then answering questions; short cases, where the candidate examines between 4 and 8 patients in quick succession and has to make a diagnosis; and a viva (oral examination). This section costs £240.
>
> Courses are available on methods of getting through the various parts of Membership and are advertised in the *BMJ*. They tend to cost between £90 and £400, depending on quality and length of course.
>
> Further information is available from the relevant Royal Colleges in London, Edinburgh and Glasgow in the UK, and Dublin in Ireland (see 'Addresses', below).

in short supply in the majority of specialties.) The time spent as an SpR varies according to specialty but is generally 4–6 years. At the end of the SpR period, a Certificate of Completion of Specialist Training (CCST) is awarded by the Joint Committee on Higher Medical Training, a body supported by the Colleges of Physicians. No exit examination is required. Further details of specialist training can be obtained from the 'Orange Book', available from the Royal College of Physicians, or from any medical school or large hospital library. Once training has been completed, a doctor is eligible for a fixed appointment as a consultant.

Medical teams are led by a consultant and consist of a varying combination of SpRs, SHOs and PRHOs. The team, or 'firm', operates in a hierarchical manner, with the most junior member performing more menial tasks. PRHOs do not generally see patients in the outpatient setting. For details of the 'double-ended sponsorship' scheme, see Box 18.2. For details of NACPME, see Box 18.3.

Box 18.2
The Overseas Doctors Training Scheme (ODTS) and 'double-ended sponsorship'

This scheme was run by the international department of the Royal College of Physicians to enable doctors trained outside the EEA to come to work in the UK. It was disbanded until further notice in 1998 owing to long waiting lists of up to 3 years. The ODTS has now been replaced by a 'double-ended sponsorship' scheme, which is also run by the College and is aimed at well-qualified doctors from overseas who have a good command of English.

A UK sponsor (based at one of the Royal Colleges) contacts a senior medical practitioner from overseas and suggests that a doctor from his or her native academic institution be recommended. If the candidate is considered suitable, the College applies for GMC registration on his or her behalf and sets up an appropriate supervised training programme, usually lasting in the order of 6–12 months. Accepted candidates are exempt from sitting the PLAB test (see p. 206), as the training programme is of a limited duration agreed in advance.

Although the UK sponsor is responsible for instigating the process and organizing registration with the GMC, financial assistance must come from the overseas doctor's native country. This is often provided by charitable trusts or national government with the idea that skills gained in the UK will then benefit local health care on the doctor's return. Overseas doctors who have come to the UK independently are not allowed to take part in this scheme, as application to a Royal College must be made by a home sponsor rather than on an individual basis.

An information sheet on the ODTS is supplied by the National Advice Centre for Postgraduate Medical Education (NACPME) at the British Council in Manchester, and information on double-ended sponsorship is available from one of the Royal Colleges in London (see 'Addresses', below).

PRACTICAL POINTS

Terms and conditions

NHS doctors are salaried and are paid for hours worked outside the 9am to 5pm working day. Part of this salary goes towards an NHS pension scheme as well as income taxation and national insurance. In February 1998, an

> **BOX 18.3**
> **NACPME**
>
> The National Advice Centre for Post-graduate Medical Education (NACPME) is based at the British Council, Manchester (see 'Addresses', below), and provides information on post-graduate medical education and training in the UK to doctors who do not possess nationality of one of the EEA member states or who qualified overseas. A number of useful information sheets are published by the British Council for EEA and non-EEA doctors wishing to work in the UK, including:
>
> - Overseas Doctors Training Scheme (ODTS)
> - Pre-Registration House Officer (PRHO) posts for overseas doctors
> - Registration requirements for overseas doctors: EEA and non-EEA
> - PLAB test and categories of exemption
> - Medical defence
> - Specialist training.

increase in doctors' salaries was announced, which was to be phased in in two stages.

Medical defence and professional disciplinary procedures

All doctors must be registered with the GMC in order to practise (see 'Registration', below) and should be insured. Hospitals do not provide medical indemnity for their employees but insurance can be obtained from organizations specializing in medical and dental defence (see 'Addresses', below). Complaints of medical negligence are referred to the GMC, where they are examined by the Committee for Professional Misconduct.

Litigation procedures differ between the private and national health (public) sector. For private treatment, the doctor must be sued personally. If the problem is caused by negligent nursing care, the private hospital is sued. For NHS treatment, it is the health authority or self-governing hospital trust that is responsible, whether the action was carried out by a senior consultant or student nurse, and this includes part-time staff. This does not mean, however, that individuals cannot be prosecuted if found culpable.

Private practice

Although the vast majority of British hospitals belong to the NHS, private health-care doctors exist. Patients insured privately pay premiums to one of over 20 private insurance organizations and can be treated either in private hospitals or in a private bed within an NHS hospital. The three principal insurance bodies are the British United Provident Association (BUPA),

Private Patients' Plan (PPP) and Western Provident Assurance. Of these organizations, which are non-profit, BUPA is the largest and has over 900 participating hospitals and around 12 000 consultants.

Only doctors at consultant level are permitted to accept care for private patients, although if these patients are admitted to an NHS hospital, the junior staff there often have to help with day-to-day management. In private hospitals, junior staff can work as locums under the admitting consultant, although these posts are generally not accredited for training purposes. Consultants working full-time in the NHS have strict conditions with respect to the amount of time spent in additional private practice.

REGISTRATION

The competent authority is the General Medical Council (GMC). The first-time registration department issues an application form which must be completed and returned, together with the necessary official documentation. Such documentation varies depending on the applicant's country of origin but generally includes the primary medical diploma, proof of nationality and a certificate of good standing, all translated into English (if applicable) by a registered translator. On requesting the application form, the applicant can also ask for details of exactly what documentation is required. A list of registered translators can be obtained from any British Council (see also 'Addresses', below). Language testing is not required for EU nationals for registration but proof of competence in English may be demanded by potential employers.

For language requirements for non-EU nationals, see Box 18.4.

BOX 18.4
IELTS and PLAB

International English Language Testing System (IELTS)
The IELTS is the chosen language test for many academic bodies in English-speaking countries including the UK, Australia, New Zealand and North America. Overseas doctors (those from outside the EEA) are required to sit this test before being considered for the PLAB test (see below).

The IELTS test consists of the four modules of reading, writing, speaking and listening. The latter two modules are uniform for all candidates. The reading and writing modules are subdivided into 'General training' or 'Academic' modules, depending on the reason for proof of proficiency in English. Doctors and other professionals aiming to work in academic institutions must sit the 'Academic' reading and writing modules. Results are available within 2 weeks of taking the test. Entrance requirements vary between institutions.

In the UK, the IELTS is developed and managed by the University of Cambridge Local Examination Syndicate (UCLES) and the British Council (see 'Addresses', below). There are test centres in over 100 countries worldwide. Addresses of these are available from the British Council in the UK or from the British Council or Embassy in the country where the test is to be taken. Further details on entering for this test are available from the Health Department at the British Council in Manchester. The British Council or British Embassy in an overseas doctor's country of origin can provide a list of dates when the examination can next be taken. In Switzerland, the British Council is in Bern (Tel: 00 41 (0)31 301 1426).

Professional and Linguistic Assessment Board (PLAB)
The PLAB test is required by all overseas (non-EEA) doctors before they are eligible to apply for GMC registration. Eligibility to sit this examination requires the following:

- medical degree awarded after the recognized training requirements by a registered academic body
- 12 months' clinical experience
- a pass in IELTS.

The original PLAB test was conducted over 2 days, with a written examination followed by a 20-minute oral examination on the second day. In April 1998, the test was extended to two parts, including a clinical examination:

- Part I consists of a written paper in three parts: multiple-choice, photographs and clinical problem-solving. It is possible to sit this first stage outside the UK, in countries in which the government has given permission for the test to be held. Currently, the only such countries are India, Pakistan and Bangladesh; Sri Lanka is in the process of obtaining permission but there is no European centre. In Britain, the test is held at one of the Royal Colleges: 14–15 times a year at the London college and once or twice a year in Scotland, in either Edinburgh or Glasgow. The pass rate is 36%.
- Part II used to consist of a 20-minute viva followed by six clinical stations but the viva was replaced in October 1998 by six additional (12 in total) clinical stations. It can be taken only in Britain, in London or Edinburgh, and takes place around ten times a year (once or twice in Edinburgh). The pass rate for candidates who sat the test between April and September in 1998 (before the introduction of the 12-station clinical exam) was 80%. The disparity between the pass rates of Parts I and II is felt to be because those who are sitting Part II are of a sufficiently high standard to have successfully sat the first stage.

Details on taking PLAB are available from the British Council in Manchester or the Royal College of Physicians of London (see 'Addresses', below). A list of courses is available from, but not endorsed by, the General Medical Council, UK.

FINDING A POST

Appointments are advertised in the *British Medical Journal (BMJ)* and *The Lancet*, which are published weekly. The classified section (a separate supplement) of the *BMJ* contains job advertisements from PRHO to consultant level and includes locum tenens appointments. All recognized posts must be advertised before being awarded and potential candidates are interviewed before a medical and non-medical panel. In order not to miss vacancies or to find out when posts are to be advertised, it is advisable to contact the medical staffing (medical personnel/human resources) department of the relevant hospital.

Locum agencies are another way of finding employment. In order to register with an agency, full GMC registration (see above) is required and a certificate of nationality, a curriculum vitae and a list of referees must be provided. Some agencies — for example, the Anaesthetists Agency (see below) — are able to find foreign postings for doctors based in Britain. It should be mentioned, though, that this agency is single-specialty, dealing only with anaesthetists, and does not specialize in overseas postings, and so jobs in other EU member states are only subject to availability.

The Association of Independent Medical Agencies (AIMA) is the UK's network of established medical agencies. Their nationwide database can be accessed by contacting any of their seven offices, of which three are listed here:

- Anaesthetists Agency — Tel: 0800 830930
- Thames Medicare — Tel: 0800 318182
- Glamorgan Medical Agency — Tel: 01685 841788

For details of work permits, see Box 18.5.

LIST OF HOSPITALS

The following is a list of hospitals which have been involved in the European Exchange Scheme. If not applying via advertisements in the medical journals, it is best to contact the medical department of the relevant hospital. Other hospital addresses are available from the British Council (see below).

United Medical and Dental Schools of Guy's and St Thomas's Hospitals
London Bridge
London SE1 9RT
Tel: 00 44 (0)171 955 4564
Fax: 00 44 (0)171 955 4230

UNITED KINGDOM

> **BOX 18.5**
> **Work permits**
>
> Overseas (non-EEA) doctors intending to seek employment in the UK, as opposed to training, require work permits. It is the duty of the prospective employer to apply for a permit on behalf of the doctor to the addresses below.
>
> **Great Britain**
> Department for Education and Employment (DFEE) Overseas Labour Service
> Moorfoot
> Sheffield S1 4PQ
> Tel: 0114 259 4074
>
> **Northern Ireland**
> Training and Employment Agency (TEA) Work Permit Branch
> Clarenden House
> 9–21 Adelaide Street
> Belfast BT2 8DJ
> Tel: 01232 871880

University of Cambridge
 Clinical School
 Hills Road
 Cambridge CB2 2QQ
 Tel: 00 44 (0)1223 336 738
 Fax: 00 44 (0)1223 336 721

St Bartholomew's Hospital
 Royal London School of Medicine and Dentistry
 West Smithfield
 London EC1A 7BE
 Tel: 00 44 (0)171 601 8342
 Fax: 00 44 (0)171 601 8505

Charing Cross Hospital
 Department of Internal Medicine
 Fulham Palace Road
 London W6 8RF
 Tel: 00 44 (0)181 846 7185
 Fax: 00 44 (0)181 846 7999

Hammersmith Hospital
 Department of Medicine (Division of Care of the Elderly Medicine)
 Du Cane Road

London W12 0HS
Tel: 00 44 (0)181 740 3958
Fax: 00 44 (0)181 743 0798

ADDRESSES

Competent authority
General Medical Council
178 Great Portland Street
London W1N 6JE
Tel: 00 44 (0)171 580 7642
Fax: 00 44 (0)171 915 2641

British Medical Association
BMA House
Tavistock Square
London WC1H 9JP
Tel: 00 44 (0)171 387 4499
Publishes the British Medical Journal. *The International Department is a good source of information.*

Royal College of Physicians of London
11 St Andrew's Place
Regent's Park
London NW1 4LE
Tel: 00 44 (0)171 935 1174
Fax: 00 44 (0)171 486 4514 (for matters regarding membership)
This college can give addresses of the other colleges.

Medical Defence Union
192 Altrincham Road
Manchester M22 4RZ
Tel: 0800 716376
One of the insurance bodies providing cover for doctors.

British Council
Examinations Business Officer
CUE
10 Spring Gardens
London SW1A 2BN
Tel: 00 44 (0)171 389 4202/4197
Fax: 00 44 (0)171 389 4140

British Council
Bridgewater House
58 Whitworth Street
Manchester M1 6BB
Tel: 00 44 (0)161 957 7000; 00 44 (0)161 957 7755 (health department); 00 44 (0)161 957 7218 (NACPME)
Fax: 00 44 (0)161 957 7111; 00 44 (0)161 957 7029 (NACPME)
There are two British Council headquarters in Britain, in London and Manchester, as well as regional centres throughout the country; only Manchester has a health department. NACPME is also based in Manchester

IELTS
IELTS Subject Officer
University of Cambridge Local Examination Syndicate
1 Hills Road
Cambridge CB1 3EU
Tel: 00 44 (0)1223 553311
Fax: 00 44 (0)1223 460278

Berlitz School of Translators
321 Oxford Street
London W1A 3BZ
Tel: 00 44 (0)171 629 7360
Fax: 00 44 (0)171 491 9158
Translations from all EU languages to English. Can be done in a matter of days, depending on subject matter. Cost depends on number of words and original language (cheapest for translations from French, Spanish and Italian). If the material to be translated is faxed with a covering letter, the school can quote a price exclusive of VAT.

REGISTRABLE QUALIFICATIONS FOR BRITISH DOCTORS GOING ABROAD

The registrable qualification granted in the United Kingdom is called the primary qualification. This is an *Approved certificate of basic knowledge*, awarded after passing a board examination of qualification, and a *Certificate of experience*, awarded by the same board, which authorizes registration as a 'fully qualified medical practitioner'. Before this stage, a doctor is eligible for partial registration.

A full list of medical schools granting registrable primary qualifications is available from the GMC. There are 15 such schools in England and Wales, 5 in Scotland and 1 in Northern Ireland. The medical school of the University of Wales is at Cardiff. The Scottish medical schools are part of the universities of Aberdeen, Dundee, Edinburgh, Glasgow and St Andrews. In Northern Ireland, the medical school is at Queen's University of Belfast. Here are some examples of the qualifications awarded in England:

- Bristol: *MB ChB Brist*
- Cambridge: *MB BChir Camb*
- London: *MB BS Lond.*

(Bachelor of Medicine and Bachelor of Surgery)

Countries in the European Economic Area: Norway, Iceland and Liechtenstein

19

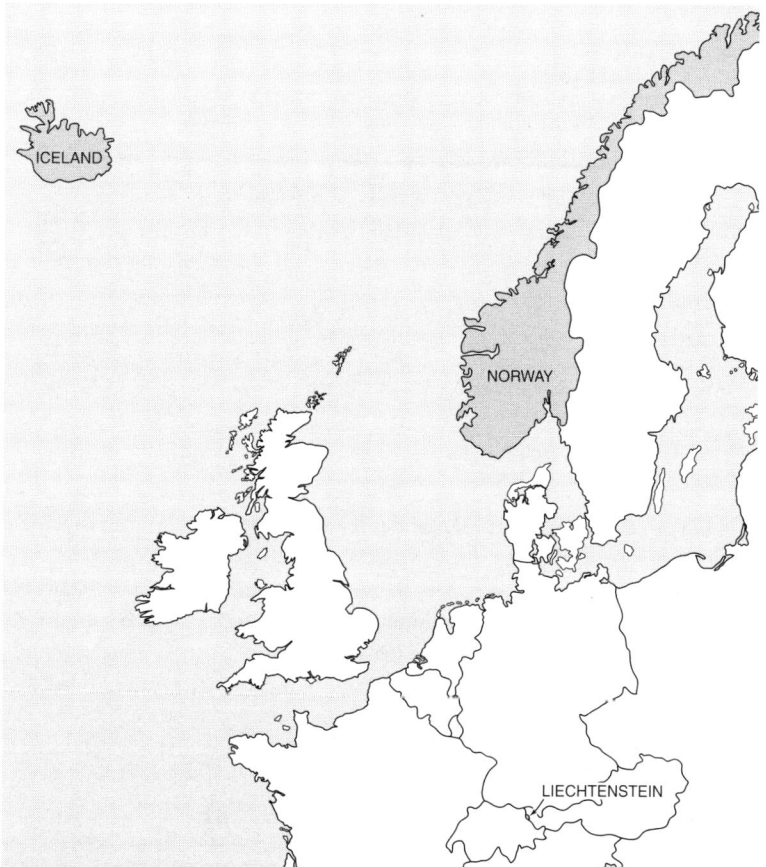

Fig. 19.1 Map showing Iceland, Norway and Liechtenstein.

Norway

Joined EFTA: 1960
Area: 324 220 km^2
Population (1998): 4.42 million
Population density: 14 persons / km^2
Language: Norwegian
Currency: Krone
Religion: Evangelical Lutheran (88%)
Government: Constitutional monarchy
GDP per head (1997): 27 400 US$
Infant mortality rate (1998): 5 deaths per 1000 live births
Average life expectancy at birth (1998): 75 (men); 81.2 (women); total 78.2 years
Unemployment (1997): 2.6%
Doctors per 10 000 population (1993): 30

BACKGROUND

Norway is a constitutional and hereditary monarchy. The King has executive power but administrative duties are carried out by the Cabinet of Ministers, headed by the Prime Minister. Legislation is dealt with by the parliament, the *Storting*. The country is divided into 19 counties, *fylker*, which are in turn divided into rural and urban municipalities, each with a governing council.

Norway's coastline in proportion to its surface area is longer than that of any other major country in the world, and over three-quarters of the 4.3 million population live within 16 km (10 miles) of the sea. The country is ethnically homogeneous, apart from several thousand Saami (Lapps) and people of Finnish origin living in the north. Almost one-third of the country lies north of the Arctic Circle but has a milder climate than one would expect owing to the North Atlantic Drift (Gulf Stream).

Education is free and compulsory in all municipalities from 7–16 years.

LANGUAGE

Norwegian is a Scandinavian language, a branch of the Germanic languages. It is most closely related to Danish for historical reasons, but is also related to Swedish.

There are two distinct dialects of Norwegian: *bokmål* ('book language', originating from the Dano-Norwegian dialect) and *nynorsk* ('new Norse', based on the dialects of rural Norway). The former is the dialect used in newspapers, television and radio, but both dialects have equal status in government institutions and schools. There is talk of merging the two to form *samnorsk*, or 'common Norwegian', but this process is not yet under way.

Norwegian uses the Danish æ and ø, which are the equivalents of Swedish ä and ö respectively. All three languages use å.

ORGANIZATION OF THE HEALTH SYSTEM

Norway runs an insurance-based health system, with contributions from employers and employees as well as from the State. Welfare benefits, including those for old age, maternity leave and disability, are provided by a compulsory National Pension Scheme.

TRAINING AND TYPES OF POST

There are four universities in Norway and each has a faculty of medicine. Nearly all institutions of higher education are financed entirely through government funds.

ADDRESSES

Competent authority
Norwegian Board of Health
Statens helsetilsyn
PO Box 8128 Dep
N-0032 Oslo
Tel: 00 47 (0)22 24 88 88
Fax: 00 47 (0)22 24 27 67

Norwegian Medical Association
Den Norske Lægeforening
PO Box 1152 Centrum
N-0107 Oslo
Tel: 00 47 (0)23 10 90 00
Fax: 00 47 (0)23 10 90 10

REGISTRABLE QUALIFICATIONS FOR NORWEGIAN DOCTORS GOING ABROAD

The registrable qualification granted in Norway is the *Bevis for bestått medisinsk embetseksamen* (Diploma of medicine), awarded by a university faculty of medicine, and a *Certificate of practical training*, issued by the competent public health authorities. The following is a list of licensing bodies (faculties of medicine) and the qualifications awarded:

- Universitetet i Bergen: *Cand Med Bergen*
- Universitetet i Oslo: *Cand Med Oslo*
- Universitetet i Tromsø: *Cand Med Tromsø*
- Universitetet i Trondheim: *Cand Med Trondheim.*

For information on Norway at medical student level, booklets are available from the following sources:

Norwegian National Academic Information Centre (NAIC)
International Education Services
University of Oslo
PO Box 1081 Blindern
N-0317 Oslo

Foreign Students Information Office (FSIO)
Langes gate 1
N-5020 Bergen
Tel: 00 47 (0)55 58 92 42

ICELAND

Joined EFTA: 1970
Area: 103, 000 km^2
Population (1998): 271 000
Population density: 2.6 persons / km^2
Language: Icelandic
Currency: Króna
Religion: Evangelical Lutheran (96%)
Government: Constitutional republic
GDP per head (1997): 21 000 US$
Infant mortality rate (1998): 5.27 deaths per 1000 live births
Average life expectancy at birth (1998): 76.8 (men); 81.1 (women); total 78.8 years
Unemployment (1997): 3.80%.

BACKGROUND

Iceland is governed under a constitution that has existed since full independence in June 1944. The Head of State is a President who is elected every 4 years. Iceland is divided into eight regions for administrative purposes. The country lies just below the Arctic Circle, around 800 km (500 miles) northwest of Scotland. As with Norway, the climate is modified favourably, in spite of its latitude, by the North Atlantic Drift (Gulf Stream).

Education is free and compulsory from ages 6–16 years.

LANGUAGE

Icelandic is a Scandinavian language. Perhaps because of the geographical isolation of Iceland, Icelandic has retained similarities to Old Norse, the language of the Vikings, which came to Iceland from Norway in the ninth century. Icelanders have avoided incorporating modern words for inventions or new concepts and such like into their language, so that words such as 'telephone', 'radio' and 'internet' have an Icelandic equivalent.

Icelandic has the letters 'eth' (ð) and 'thorn' (þ), seen in Old English, as well as the æ seen in Danish and Norwegian.

TRAINING AND TYPES OF POST

Medical studies as an undergraduate are of 6 years' duration. On passing final examinations, the student is awarded the professional degree known as the *Kandidat*. The graduate then has to complete 1 year of practical training before being eligible for full registration.

There are three universities in Iceland, although only one, the University of Iceland in Reykjavik, has a faculty of medicine. This is the oldest and largest university, founded in 1911.

ADDRESSES

Competent authority
Ministry of Health and Social Security
Heibrigdisraduneyti
Laugavegi 116
150 Reykjavik
Tel: 00 354 (0)560 9700
Fax: 00 354 (0)551 9165
E-mail: postur@htr.tjr.is

Icelandic Embassy
1 Eaton Terrace
London SW1W 8EY
Tel: 0171 730 1683

University of Iceland
International Office
Vid-Sud-urgötu
101 Reykjavik
Tel: 00 354 (0)525 4311
Fax: 00 354 (0)525 4723

REGISTRABLE QUALIFICATIONS FOR ICELANDIC DOCTORS GOING ABROAD

The registrable qualification granted in Iceland is the *Próf i læknisfræði fra læknadeild Háskóla Islands* (Diploma awarded by the University of Iceland faculty of medicine) and a *Certificate of practical training* of at least 12 months in a hospital, issued by the Chief Medical Officer. The licensing body and qualification awarded are as follows:

- Háskóla Islands Læknadeild: *Cand Med et Chir Reykjavik.*

LIECHTENSTEIN

Joined EFTA: 1995
Area: 160 km^2
Population (1998): 31 700
Population density: 198 persons / km^2
Language: German
Currency: Swiss franc
Religion: Roman Catholic (80%): Protestant (7%)
Government: Hereditary constitutional monarchy
GDP per head (1996): 23 000 US$
Infant mortality rate (1998): 5.28 deaths per 1000 live births
Average life expectancy at birth (1994): 75.5 (men); 80.5 (women); total 78 years
Unemployment (1997): 1.6%

BACKGROUND

Liechtenstein is one of the smallest independent states in the world, sandwiched between Switzerland and Austria. The principality is a hereditary constitutional monarchy. Approximately 4% of national income is from the sale of postage stamps. The other important source of income is from exported goods, particularly pharmaceuticals and false teeth.

LANGUAGE

German is the official language of Liechtenstein (see Chapter 9).

TRAINING AND TYPES OF POST

There are two small institutions of higher education but no universities and therefore no faculty of medicine. Students from Liechtenstein usually go to Switzerland or Austria for higher education under the terms of special agreements negotiated by the Liechtenstein government.

ADDRESSES

For further information, contact:

Department of Education
Schulamt des Fürstentums Liechtenstein
Herrengasse 2
FL-9490 Vaduz
Liechtenstein
Tel: 00 41 (0)75 236 61 11

REGISTRABLE QUALIFICATIONS FOR DOCTORS FROM LIECHTENSTEIN GOING ABROAD

Qualifications required for medical registration are the *Diplomas, certificates and other titles* awarded in another State to which Directive 93/16/EEC applies and which are listed in Article 3 of that Directive, together with a *Certificate of completed practical training*, issued by the State's competent authority.

Switzerland

20

Area: 41 293 km^2
Population (1998): 7.26 million
Population density: 176 persons / km^2
Languages: French (18%); German (65%); Italian (10%); Romansch (< 1%)
Currency: Swiss franc
Religion: Roman Catholic (46%); Protestant (40%)
Government: Federal republic
GDP per head (1997): 23 800 US$
Health expenditure as % of GDP (1995): 9.8%
Infant mortality rate (1998): 4.92 deaths per 1000 live births
Average life expectancy at birth: 75.7 (men); 82.2 (women); total 78.9 years
Unemployment (1997): 5%
Doctors per 10 000 population (1994): 31

BACKGROUND

Switzerland is a mountainous federal republic in west-central Europe. Over 70% of its area is covered by the Alps and water power is the chief national resource. Although Bern is the capital, the largest city is Zürich and Geneva is the cultural and financial centre. The country has a well-developed industrialized economy and a very high standard of living.

National executive power is vested in a Federal Council or *Bundesrat*, whose seven members are elected every 4 years. Legislative power is vested in the Swiss parliament, which is called the Federal Assembly. Switzerland is a confederation of 23 states or *cantons*, of which three are subdivided into half-*cantons* for administrative purposes. *Cantons* have elected executive and legislative councils which deal with matters not delegated to the confederation. Women gained the right to vote in local and cantonal elections in most areas in the 1970s. In Appenzell, this right was awarded to women only in 1990.

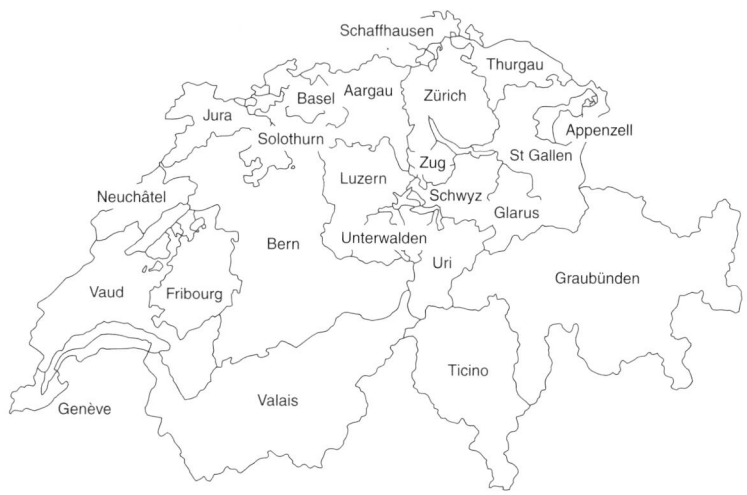

Fig. 20.1 Map of Switzerland.

In December 1992, a referendum in Switzerland led to the rejection of proposals to establish a European Economic Area (EEA) and the country has subsequently never joined the EU. Swiss citizens do not therefore enjoy the freedom of movement and mutual recognition of professional qualifications that exists between citizens of EU member states. Consequently, non-Swiss nationals considering employment in Switzerland require a work permit and a residence permit, both of which are valid for 1 year. Application for these permits is the responsibility of the future employer.

Switzerland is still, however, a popular destination for doctors seeking employment in French- or German-speaking institutions and the standard of medicine is considered high. Two hospitals have been involved in the European Exchange Scheme, as listed later in this chapter.

LANGUAGE

Romansch, one of the three Rhaeto-Romanic languages (members of the Romance family), is spoken by around 50 000 people in the Swiss canton of Graubünden (Grisons), bordering Austria and Italy. Although this amounts to only 1% of the population, Romansch is one of Switzerland's four official languages, along with French, German and Italian.

In a minority of cantons, the most commonly spoken language is Schwyzertutsch or Swiss German, which is an Allemanic dialect of, and very different from, 'standard' German (see Chapter 9).

ORGANIZATION OF THE HEALTH SYSTEM

Health care in Switzerland is based on compulsory insurance. One of the criticisms of the present system is that there are minimal cost constraints, so that hospitals with available facilities can perform frequent investigations in the knowledge that they will be reimbursed by insurance bodies. This has the effect of increasing insurance premiums for those in employment and could cause difficulties in the future. Old age and disability benefits are financed by a payroll tax on both employers and employees. Unemployment insurance became compulsory in 1976.

TRAINING AND TYPES OF POST

Medical training in Switzerland is broadly similar to that in other countries in Europe, with an undergraduate period of 6 years followed by general and then specialist training. The titles used for grades of hospital doctor are as for francophone or German-speaking institutions in other countries:

- Following qualification, the junior doctor is an *Assistantartz / assistant(e)* for 6 years, which involves training in general internal medicine followed by training in the chosen specialty. Although there is no MRCP equivalent, there is a post-graduate examination but passing it does not seem to be required in order to progress up the career ladder.
- After specialty training has been completed, the doctor becomes an *Oberartz*. The equivalent terms in French would be a *résident(e)* or a *chef de clinique*, depending on seniority. In German-speaking academic hospitals, an *Oberartz* has a contract to practise for a fixed duration, usually around 8 years. At the end of this period, if the doctor is not then promoted within the system — for example, to the level of professor — he or she has to leave the post. The options then are to find an equivalent post in a peripheral hospital or else to engage in private practice.

There is no equivalency of training or specialist status between Switzerland and EU member states and so a non-Swiss doctor wishing to practise full-time as a specialist in Switzerland has to retrain. A language test is also usually required. The advantage of the European Exchange Scheme is that these problems can be bypassed. The junior doctor posts in the scheme have been developed specifically for exchange candidates and, because the exchange institutions have longstanding contact with those in EU countries and the posts are short-term (6–12 months), no formal 'equivalence of training' procedure is required.

FINDING A POST (OUTSIDE THE EXCHANGE SCHEME)

Vacant posts are advertised weekly in the *Bulletin of Swiss Physicians*, published by:

Hans Huber AG,
Länggassstrasse 76,
CH-3000 Bern 9

or in the *Swiss Medical Journal* (*Schweizerische Ärztezeitung*):

Verlag Huber & Co AG
Zeughausgasse 22
CH-3011 Bern
Tel: 00 41 31 22 93 31

LIST OF HOSPITALS

The two hospitals listed here are those which have taken part in the European Exchange Scheme:

Hôpital Cantonal Universitaire (*French-speaking*)
Clinique de Médecine I
24 rue Micheli-du-Crest
1211 Genève 4
Tel: 00 41 (0)22 372 9052
Fax: 00 41 (0)22 372 9116

Kantonsspital Basel (*German-speaking*)
Medizinische Universitätsklinik B
Petersgraben 4
4031 Basel
Tel: 00 41 (0)61 265 4292
Fax: 00 41 (0)61 265 5390

ADDRESSES

Swiss Medical Association
Verbinding der Schweizer Ärzte
(Foederatio Medicorum Helveticorum – FMH)
Elfenstrasse 18
CH-3000 Bern 16
Tel: 00 41 (0)31 351 5543
Fax: 00 41 (0)31 351 55770

SWITZERLAND

Federal Office of Public Health
Medical Professional Examinations Sections
Bollwerk 27
Mail Box 2644
CH-3001 Bern

Cantonal health authorities

Central Office
Schweizerische Sanitätsdirektoren-Konferenz
Conférence des directeurs cantonaux des affaires sanitaires
Terrassenweg 18
3012 Bern
Tel: 00 41 (0)31 301 2152
Fax: 00 41 (0)31 301 22363

In Basel (*German-speaking*)
Sanitätsdepartement
St Alban-Vorstadt 25
4006 Basel
Tel: 00 41 (0)61 267 8181

In Geneva (*French-speaking*)
Département de la Santé Publique
Case postale 684
1211 Genève 3
Tel: 00 41 (0)22 319 2906
Fax: 00 41 (0)22 320 9965

In Ticino (*Italian-speaking*)
Dipartimento delle opere sociali
Residenza governativa
6501 Bellinzona
Tel: 00 41 (0)92 24 38 65

National formulary

Bréviaire des Médicaments
Documed SA
Case postale 217
4020 Bâle
Tel: 00 41 (0)61 311 8866
Fax: 00 41 (0)61 311 0252
This is a pocket edition of the Swiss Compendium of Medicines. *Drugs are listed in alphabetical order, rather than according to class.*

SWISS DOCTORS WORKING IN BRITAIN

Swiss graduates may apply for limited GMC registration. As Switzerland is not part of the EEA, Swiss nationals must sit the PLAB test (see p. 206) before they are eligible to register. The process for registration is as described for overseas doctors in Chapter 18.

In special circumstances, exemption from sitting the PLAB test may be obtained. This would apply either to Swiss nationals who have trained in an EU member state or to doctors native of a member state who have trained in Switzerland. Royal College Sponsorship of candidates taking part in the European Exchange Scheme is another means of obtaining exemption. The best approach is to contact the international department of the Royal College of Physicians to see how best to proceed.

If the PLAB test is not required, the doctor must obtain an LR3 form, which is issued by either one of the Royal Colleges or the academic institution at which the doctor has been accepted for employment. The route to obtaining registration for doctors exempt from sitting PLAB is as follows:

1. Application to the appropriate Royal College in Britain with details of the proposed appointment to obtain an LR3 form. The original certificates of primary qualification (with certified English translation) are required, together with a fee of £400.

2. The LR3 form is then forwarded to the prospective employer for endorsement and for a copy of the prospective job description. If the job description is approved by the Royal College, the final section of the LR3 relating to sponsorship can be completed and submitted, together with qualification documentation, to the GMC for processing and registration.

3. Note that a language test may still be required, organized by the British Council. There is also a requirement of 3 years' post-graduate training (in the candidate's native Switzerland) before applications can be considered.